Prentice Hall Health

complete review

ᴼᶠ Dental Assisting

Emily Andujo, RDH, BS, MS
Dental Hygeine Education
Pima Community College
Tucson, Arizona

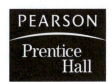

PEARSON

Prentice
Hall

Upper Saddle River, New Jersey 07458

Library of Congress Cataloging-in-Publication Data

Andujo Emily.
  Prentice Hall Health's outline review of dental assisting/Emily
Andujo
    p. ; cm.
Includes bibliographical references and index.
  ISBN 0-13-088350-6
  1. Dental assistants—Examinations, questions, etc. 2.
Dentistry—Examinations, questions, etc.
  [DNLM: 1. Dental Care—Examination Questions. 2. Dental
Assistants--education. WU 18.2 A577p 2004] I. Title: Complete review
of dental assisting. II. Title.
  RK60.5 .A533 2004
  617.6'0233--dc21
                                             2003010983

Publisher: Julie Levin Alexander
Assistant to Publisher: Regina Bruno
Acquisitions Editor: Mark Cohen
Assistant Editor: Melissa Kerian
Editorial Assistant: Mary Ellen Ruitenberg
Marketing Manager: Nicole Benson
Channel Marketing Manager: Rachele Strober
Director of Production and Manufacturing:
  Bruce Johnson
Managing Production Editor: Patrick Walsh
Production Liaison: Alexander Ivchenko

Production Editor: Jessica Balch, Pine Tree Composition
Manufacturing Manager: Ilene Sanford
Manufacturing Buyer: Pat Brown
Design Director: Cheryl Asherman
Design Coordinator: Maria Guglielmo-Walsh
Cover and Interior Designer: Janice Bielawa
Composition: Pine Tree Composition, Inc.
Manager of Media Production: Amy Peltier
New Media Project Manager: Stephen Hartner
Printing and Binding: Banta Book Group
Cover Printer: Phoenix Color Corp.

Pearson Education, Ltd., *London*
Pearson Education Australia Pty. Limited, *Sydney*
Pearson Education Singapore Pte. Ltd.
Pearson Education North Asia Ltd., *Hong Kong*
Pearson Education Canada, Ltd., *Toronto*
Pearson Educación de Mexico, S.A. de C.V.
Pearson Education—Japan, *Tokyo*
Pearson Education Malaysia, Pte. Ltd.
Pearson Education, Upper Saddle River, New Jersey

10 9 8 7 6 5 4 3 2 1
ISBN 0-13-088350-6

*This book is dedicated
to all dental assistants and
dental assisting students who aspire to
excel in their chosen profession.*

Contents

Preface / vi
Acknowledgments / vii
Contributors / viii
Reviewers / x
Introduction / xi

1 Introduction to the Dental Assisting Certification Exam / 1
2 Biomedical Sciences / 13
3 Dental Anatomy / 31
4 Preventive Dentistry / 47
5 Chairside Assisting / 59
6 Dental Radiology / 71
7 Dental Materials / 99
8 Infection Control / 113
9 Occupational Safety / 127
10 Medical Emergencies / 147
11 Dental Practice Management / 163
12 Simulated Comprehensive Exam / 177

Glossary / 189
Bibliography / 193
Resources / 197
Index / 199

Preface

Prentice Hall Health's Complete Review of Dental Assisting is designed to act as a study companion for students who are (1) preparing for national board examinations and/or (2) pursuing self-assessment in dental assisting. This book enables the reader to review relevant material through the use of interactive technology to assist you to gain more practice and review while becoming familiar with the types of questions given on board examinations. This exam preparation review book serves as an adjunct to regular dental science course work. The review book should be a supplement to the fundamental aspects of dental assisting knowledge.

Prentice Hall Health's Complete Review of Dental Assisting is designed in an easy-to-use outline format followed by sample practice test questions with answers and rationales. As an added feature, the companion CD-ROM and links to the Prentice Hall Web site study system revolutionizes exam preparation. The World Wide Web provides links to numerous dental sites that will serve as additional resources and access to libraries all over the world.

We wish you well in your dental assisting professional careers and hope this text provides additional benefits of examination success for your future professional career endeavors.

Acknowledgments

I would like to thank Mark Cohen, Senior Editor of Health Professions at Prentice Hall, for his continued support and commitment to the integration of interactive technology for the *Success Across the Boards Review Series* exam preparation books. I would also like to acknowledge Melissa Kerian, Assistant Editor at Prentice Hall, and Martha Currise, who provided guidance and support during the development of this book.

I would like to thank Kettil Gunnberg, photographer and audio video technician, and Tami Guido, dental hygiene student at Pima Community College, for their contributions to this text.

Thank you to my friends, colleagues, and contributors for their suggestions and encouragement—in particular to Dr. Ronald Flores and the Saint Elizabeth of Hungary dental staff. Additional thanks to Olivia Ordonez, CDA, dental office manager and safety coordinator, and Suzette Portillo, dental receptionist and manuscript typist.

A special note of thanks to my computer mentor and soul mate for the extra patience displayed and the countless hours spent formatting, inputting digital photos, and editing this project to final perfection for copy. Thanks, "D."

Emily Andujo

Contributors

Stephanie Dante, CDA, RDA, AS
Instructor, Dental Practice Management
Department of Dental Assisting
Cerritos Community College
Norwalk, California
Dental Management-First Edition

Joleen Failor, CDA, RDA, BVE
Director, Department of Dental
  Assisting
Division of Health Occupations
Cerritos Community College
Norwalk, California
Chairside Assisting-First Edition

Robert Hankel, DDS
Dental Management Consultant
Dental Practice Broker
Adjunct Faculty
Pima Community College
Tucson, Arizona
Dental Management-First Edition

Adelle Krayer, RDH, BA, MA
Assistant Professor
Dental Hygiene Department
Cerritos College
Lecturer, University California
  Los Angeles
Infection Control & OSHA Compliance
  Consultant
Infection Control-First Edition
Occupational Safety

Richard J. Nagy, DDS, BA
Director, Department of Periodontics
Veterans Administration Medical Center
  West Los Angeles
Lecturer, University of California,
  Los Angeles, School of Dentistry
Los Angeles, California
Staff Dentist
Rancho Los Amigos Hospital
Downey, California
Biomedical Sciences—Oral Pathology
Medical Emergencies-First Edition

Joan Otomo-Corgel, DDS, MPH
Adjunct Assistant Professor
Department of Periodontics
University of California, Los Angeles,
  School of Dentistry
Los Angeles, California
Faculty, Staff Dentist
Veterans Administration Medical Center,
  West Los Angeles
Staff Dentist
Rancho Los Amigos Hospital
Downey, California
Preventive Dentistry
Biomedical Sciences—Pharmacology,
  Oral Pathology
Chairside Assisting—Periodontics-First
  Edition

Virginia F. Santos, CDA, RDA, BVE
Director, Department of Dental Assisting
  (Retired)
Division of Health Science
East Los Angeles Occupational Center
Los Angeles, California
*Chairside Assisting—Orthodontics-First
  Edition*

Edward F. Sparks, DDS, PC
General Practice Dentist
Clinical Adjunct Faculty
Department of Dental Hygiene
  Educatiion
Pima Community College
Tucson, Arizona
Infection Control-Second Edition

**Jane M. Watanabe, CDA, RDA,
OSMA, MSEd**
Administrative Coordinator, Oral and
  Maxillofacial Surgery
Surgical Assistant for Implant Program
Former Coordinator Department of
  Auxiliary Utilization
University of Southern California School
  of Dentistry
Los Angeles, California
*Chairside Assisting—Oral and Maxillo-
  facial Surgery-First Edition*

Donna J. Wedell, CDA, RDA, AS
Instructor, Radiology and Dental Science
  Department of Dental Assisting
Cerritos Community College
Norwalk, California
Dental Radiology-First Edition

Sheila D. Whetstone, RDH, BHS
Medical Education Program Coordinator
Veterans Administration Medical Center
Long Beach, California
Dental Radiology-First Edition

Rizkalla Zakhaty, PhD
Associate Professor of Anatomy (Retired)
Department of Basic Sciences
University of Southern California School
  of Dentistry
Los Angeles, California
General Anatomy
Dental Anatomy-First Edition

Reviewers

Marsha E. Bower, CDA, RDH, MA
Assistant Professor
Dental Studies
Monroe Community College
Rochester, New York

Shelby Chadwick, CDA, BS, M.Ed.
Dental Instructor
Coastal Carolina Community College
Jacksonville, North Carolina

Lydia Duffey, RDH, BHS
Assistant Professor
Dental Health Services Department
Palm Beach Community College
Lake Worth, Florida

Nancy Zinser, RDH, MS
Professor and Chair
Dental Health Services
Palm Beach Community College
Lake Worth, Florida

Introduction

 SUCCESS ACROSS THE BOARDS:
THE PRENTICE HALL HEALTH REVIEW SERIES

Prentice Hall is pleased to present *Success Across the Boards,* our new review series. These authoritative texts give you expert help in preparing for certifying examinations. Each title in the series comes with its own technology package, including a CD-ROM and a Companion Website. You will find that this powerful combination of text and media provides you with expert help and guidance for achieving success across the boards. This outline review for the dental assistant provides help for preparing for the Certified Dental Assistant Examinations in General Chairside, Infection Control, Radiation Health and Safety, Certified Orthodontic Assistant, and Certified Dental Practice Management Administrator.

COMPONENTS OF THE SERIES

The series is made up of one book and CD combination, as well as a Companion Website that supports the book.

About the Book: Complete Review of Dental Assisting by Emily Andujo

- *Outline Content Review:* Key topics that may be covered on the board examinations are included in this book. With the easy-to-use summary box format, you can quickly identify the important ideas, concepts, and facts that are presented. Important terms are defined where necessary, and illustrations are included where they will help illuminate and clarify information. The concept of the review book is to make it easier to understand information you have learned elsewhere—in courses, from textbooks, in the field. The purpose of the summary boxes is to help you focus your review on the most important information and use your study time most effectively.

- *Study Questions:* Multiple choice questions at the end of each chapter follow the format of questions that appear on the examination. Working through these questions after reviewing each chapter will help you assess your strengths and weaknesses in each topic of study. Correct answers and comprehensive rationales are included.

About the CD-ROM

A CD-ROM is included in the back of this book. The CD provides additional practice multiple choice questions, additional full-color illustrations (photos) to help illuminate and clarify information, and an audio glossary.

- *Practice Questions:* The accompanying CD includes over 300 stand-alone questions. The software was designed so that you can practice by topic or through simulated exams. Correct answers and comprehensive rationales follow all questions. You will receive immediate feedback to identify your strengths and weaknesses in each topic covered.

- *Audio Glossary:* Over 200 words are pronounced and definitions provided to help you review and practice the all-important terms you need to know.

Companion Website for Dental Assisting Review

Visit the companion website at **www.prenhall.com/ review** for Specialty Examination Practice Tests in Dental Practice Management Administration and Orthodontic Assisting. The companion website also has additional information about the exam, and links to related resources. Designed as a supplement to the review text you will want to bookmark this site and return frequently for the most current information on your path to success.

CERTIFICATION

By becoming DANB certified, dental assistants demonstrate their commitment to excellence. Maintaining a DANB credential shows personal professional growth and commitment to quality dental care.

ABOUT THE CERTIFIED DENTAL ASSISTANT EXAMINATIONS

DANB is the recognized certification and credentialing agency for dental assistants. The American Dental Association recognizes DANB as the certification agency for dental assistants.

The DANB CDA and/or Radiation Health and Safety (RHS) and Infection Control (ICE) examinations are required or recognized as meeting regulatory requirements in over thirty states. The exam is comprehensive and consists of three components. The candidate must meet minimum performance standards in each component to earn CDA certification. There are three components of this exam: Radiation Health and Safety (RHS), which consists of 100 multiple-choice items, Infection Control Examination (ICE), which consists of 100 multiple-choice items, and General Chairside (GC), which consists of 120 multiple-choice items.

The written format of the examination is given three times a year. The computerized format of the DANB exam allows the candidates more flexibility in scheduling dates and times. There are no specific examination dates nor application deadlines for the computerized format of the DANB exam.

Additional information about the test may be obtained by contacting the Dental Assisting National Board, Inc. (DANB), 676 N. St. Clair Street, Suite 1880, Chicago, Illinois 60611 or by calling 1-800-FOR-DANB or 312-642-3368. Fax 312-642-1475, Web site **www.danb.org** and e-mail address danbmail@danb.org.

STUDY TIPS

Review Materials

Choose review materials that contain the information you need to study. Save time by making sure you aren't studying anything needlessly. For preparation before the exam, the best study preparation would be to use both the Review Book and the CD-ROM. Use the references in these review materials to easily find related textbooks and resource websites if additional study is required. We strongly encourage all exam candidates to obtain a copy of the DANB Task Analysis for the component examinations of the Certified Dental Assistant (CDA), Radiation Health and Safety (RHS), Infection Control Examination (ICE), Certified Orthodontic Assistant (COA), and Certified Dental Practice Management Administrator (CDPMA).

Set a Study Schedule

Use your time-management skills to set a schedule that will help you feel as prepared as you can be. Consider all the relevant factors—the materials you need to study, how many months, weeks, or days until the test date, and how much time you can study each day. If you establish your schedule ahead of time and write it in your date book, you will be much more likely to follow it.

Take Practice Tests

Practice as much as possible, using the questions at the end of each chapter in this book, along with over 400 more questions available in the accompanying CD, and the Companion Website. These questions were designed to follow the format of the exam, so the more you practice with these questions, the better prepared you will be on test day.

The practice tests on the CD will give you a chance to experience the exam before you actually have to take it and will also let you know how you're doing and where you need to do better. For best results, we recommend you take a practice test two to three weeks before you are scheduled to take the actual exam. Spend the next weeks targeting those areas in which you performed poorly by reviewing the chapter outlines and practicing additional questions in those areas.

Practice under test-like conditions—in a quiet room, with no books or notes to help you, and with a clock to monitor the time limit. Try to come as close as you can to duplicating the actual test situation.

TAKING THE EXAMINATION

Prepare Physically

When taking the examination, you need to work efficiently under time pressure. If your body is tired or under stress, you might not think as clearly or perform as well as you usually do. If you can, avoid staying up all night. Get some sleep so you wake up rested and alert.

Eating right is also important. The best advice is to eat a light, well-balanced meal before a test. When time is short, grab a quick-energy snack such as a banana, orange juice, or a granola bar.

The Examination Site

The examination site should be located prior to the required examination time. One suggestion is to find the site and parking facilities the day before the test. Parking fee information should be obtained so sufficient money can be taken along on the examination day.

Allow plenty of time for travel to the site in case of unexpected mishaps such as traffic snarls. During travel, think positive thoughts (e.g., "My preparation for the exam was thorough, so I'll be able to answer the questions easily."). Maintain a confident attitude to prevent unnecessary stress.

Materials

Be sure to take all required identification materials, registration forms, and any other items required by the testing organization or center. Read information and instructions supplied by the testing organizations thoroughly to be sure you have all necessary materials before the day of the exam.

Read Test Directions

Read the examination directions thoroughly! Because some board examinations have different test sections with different question formats, it is important to be aware of changes in directions. Read each set of directions completely before starting a new section of questions.

Machine-scored tests require you use a special pencil to fill in a small box on a computerized answer sheet. Use the right pencil (usually a number 2), and mark your answers in the correct space. Neatness counts on these tests, because the computer can misread stray pencil marks or partially erased answers. Periodically check the answer number against the question number to make sure they match. One question skipped can cause every answer following it to be marked incorrectly.

If choosing the computerized format for testing purposes, be sure to follow the directions at the testing site for use of the computer. Steps for taking the test on the computer and how to indicate your answer choice should be provided for you.

Selecting the Right Answer

Keep in mind only one answer is correct. First read the stem of the question with *each* possible choice provided and eliminate choices that are obviously incorrect. Be cautious about choosing the first answer that *might* be correct; all possibilities should be considered before the final choice is made; the best answer should be selected.

If a question is complicated, try to break it down into small sections that are easy to understand. Pay special attention to qualifiers such as *only, except,* etc. For example, negative words in a question can confuse your understanding of what the question asks ("Which of the following is not. . .").

Intelligent Guessing

If you don't know the answer, eliminate those answers that you know or suspect are wrong. Your goal is to narrow down your choices. Here are some questions to ask yourself:

- Is the choice accurate in its own terms? If there's an error in the choice—for example, a term that is incorrectly defined—the answer is wrong.

- Is the choice relevant? An answer may be accurate, but it may not relate to the essence of the question.
- Are there any distractors, such as *always, never, all, none,* or *every?* Qualifiers make it easy to find an exception that makes a choice incorrect.

Mark answers you aren't sure of, and go back to them at the end of the test. Ask yourself whether you would make the same guesses again. Chances are you will leave your answers alone, but you may notice something that will make you change your mind—a qualifier that affects meaning or a remembered fact that will enable you to answer the question without guessing.

Watch the Clock

Keep track of how much time is left and how you are progressing. Wearing a watch may be helpful. You will be notified by the test proctor throughout the examination when you are at the halfway point, as well as how much time is remaining. Some students are so concerned about time, they rush through the exam and have time left over. In such situations, it's easy to leave early. The best approach, however, is to take your time. Stay until the end so that you can check your answers.

KEYS TO SUCCESS ACROSS THE BOARDS

- Study, review, and practice
- Keep a positive, confident attitude
- Follow all directions on the examination
- Do your best

Good luck!

You are encouraged to visit http://www.prenhall.com/success *for additional tips on studying, test-taking, and other keys to success. At this stage of your education and career you will find these tips helpful.*

Some of the study and test-taking tips were adapted from **Keys to Effective Learning,** *2nd Ed. by Carol Carter, Joyce Bishop, and Sarah Lyman Kravits.*

CHAPTER

1

Introduction to the Dental Assisting Certification Examination
Preparation, Format, and Strategies

contents

➤ Administration of the Examination

➤ Eligibility Requirements

➤ Testing Candidates With a Disability Condition

➤ Testing Schedule

➤ Examination Format

➤ Distribution of Items

➤ Types of Questions

➤ Multiple-Choice Test Strategies

➤ Test Anxiety

➤ Examination Scoring

➤ Physical Conditions

Certification examinations are available for advancement and growth within the dental assisting profession. As you approach the beginning of a career in dental assisting you will discover that to promote the practice of quality dental assisting the designated certification examinations in Chairside Assisting, Radiation Health and Safety, Infection Control, Orthodontic Assisting, and Dental Practice Management Administration will allow you to continue to learn and grow professionally.

This chapter is intended for dental assisting students who are preparing to take the Certified Dental Assisting examinations and for working dental assistants who are seeking professional advancement within their chosen careers.

A major component of success for passing any examination is familiarity with the test itself. This chapter—Preparing for the Dental Assisting Certification Examinations—presents the reader with practical information about the examination, as well as helpful study hints, methods to develop a positive attitude, and strategies for overcoming test anxiety. All of these elements are essential to successfully passing the Certification examinations.

➤ ADMINISTRATION OF THE EXAMINATION

The Dental Assisting National Board, Inc. (DANB) is the nationally recognized certification and credentialing agency for dental assistants. DANB is a member of the National Organization for Competency Assurance (NOCA). The National Commission for Certifying Agencies, a NOCA Commission with responsibility for evaluating credentialing programs has accredited DANB and found the certification and credentialing agency to meet its highest standards, thus helping to assure validity, reliability, and objectivity in the testing process.

DANB's nine-member Board of Directors represents the American Dental Association, American Dental Assistants Association, American Dental Education Association, American Association of Dental Examiners, DANB Certificants, and The Public. The dental assisting certification national board examinations are given for professional advancement, to demonstrate the dental assistant's knowledge, and to promote quality dental assisting practices.

➤ ELIGILBILITY REQUIREMENTS

To take the Certified Dental Assisting Examination candidates must submit an application to DANB and document their eligibility in order to qualify for a certification exam. Eligibility may be determined by several identified pathways as outlined in the *Certified Dental Assistant Candidate's Guide,* which may be obtained from the Dental Assisting National Board. Inc. 676 N. St. Clair Street, Suite 1880, Chicago, Illinois 60611 (1-800-FOR-DANB). Web site address: www.danb.org.

➤ TESTING CANDIDATES WITH A DISABILITY CONDITION

DANB adheres to the provisions of the Americans with Disabilities Act. Refer to the *Certified Dental Assistant Candidate's Guide* for further information and a copy of the *Special Accommodations Request Form,* which is to be submitted with the application. DANB examinations are only administered in the English language.

➤ TESTING SCHEDULE

The examination dates and application deadlines are listed in the *Certified Dental Assistant Candidate's Guide.* The candidates must select to take the examination in either a written paper-and-pencil format or in a computerized format. The computerized format of the examination is scheduled throughout the year. There are no specific examination dates nor application deadlines for the computerized format.

The written format is usually scheduled three times a year and at designated locations. This particular format will be offered only through the end of the 2003 year cycle. Both formats of the examination are proctored by trained examiners.

➤ EXAMINATION FORMAT

The Certified Dental Assistant Examination has three components: General Chairside, Radiation Health & Safety, and Infection Control. There are 120 test items on the General Chairside exam, 100 test items on the Radiation Health & Safety exam, and 100 test items on the Infection Control component. Candidates are given 4 hours to complete the full 320-item Certified Dental Assistant Examination.

Candidates who only take a single component of the three-part certification exam will have 1½ hours for the General Chairside component, 1¼ hours for the Radiation Health & Safety component, and 1¼ hours for the Infection Control component.

The Certified Orthodontic Assistant (COA) examination contains two components. There are 200 test items on Orthodontic Assisting and 100 test items on Infection Control. Candidates may take the full 300 question examination or either component in any order. The Infection Control component requires 1¼ hours to complete. The Orthodontic Assisting component has 200 questions and would require approximately 2¾ hours.

The Certified Dental Practice Management Administrator (CDPMA) examination contains test items from both the Radiation Health & Safety and Infection Control components of the Certified General Chairside examination.

➤ DISTRIBUTION OF ITEMS

The **Certified Dental Assisting Examination** consists of three components; General Chairside, Radiation Health and Safety, and Infection Control. The distribution of items is approximately as outlined below:

I. GENERAL CHAIRSIDE COMPONENT (contains 120 multiple-choice items)
   A. Collection and recording of clinical data (9%)
   B. Chairside dental procedures (48%)
   C. Chairside dental materials (11%)
   D. Lab materials and procedures (4%)
   E. Patient education and oral health management (9%)
   F. Prevention and management of emergencies (13%)
   G. Office management procedures (6%)

II. RADIATION HEALTH AND SAFETY COMPONENT (contains 100 multiple-choice items)
   A. Expose and evaluate intraoral and extraoral radiographs (37%)
   B. Processing procedures (12%)
   C. Mounting/labeling (11%)
   D. Radiation safety—patient (23%)
   E. Radiation safety—operator (11%)
   F. Storage and disposal (2%)
   G. Quality assurance (4%)

III. INFECTION CONTROL COMPONENT (contains 100 multiple-choice items)
   A. Collection and recording of data (10%)
   B. Patient and dental health care worker education (10%)
   C. Prevent cross-contamination and transmission (20%)
   D. Maintain aseptic conditions (10%)
   E. Select disinfection or sterilization (5%)
   F. Perform sterilization procedures (15%)
   G. Perform disinfection procedures (10%)
   H. Occupational safety (20%)

IV. SPECIALTY EXAMINATIONS for the Orthodontic Assisting and Dental Practice Management Administrator each have components which contain content material from the Certified Dental Assisting Examination components.

➤ TYPES OF QUESTIONS

The certification examination includes three different question formats: *one best answer—single item, negative format,* and *matching.* In some cases, a group of questions may be related to a dental charting exercise or dental condition for interpretation. Some of the items are stated in the negative. In such instances, the negative word is in capital letters (e.g., "All of the following are correct EXCEPT," "Which of the following choices is NOT correct?" *and* "Which of the following is LEAST correct?"). Additionally, some questions have illustrative material (instruments, x-rays, tables) that will require further understanding and interpretation on your part.

One Best Answer—Single-Item Question

This type of question presents a problem or asks a question and is followed by four choices, only one of which is entirely correct. The directions preceding this type of question generally will appear as follows.

DIRECTIONS (Question 1): Each of the questions or incomplete statements in this section is followed by four suggested answers or completions. Select the ONE lettered answer or completion that is BEST in each case.

1. The most important reason for using alginate for preliminary impressions is the
   A. pleasant color and taste of the material.
   B. speed and simplicity of mixing.
   C. ability of alginate to withstand the pouring of multiple models from a single impression.
   D. greater precision of alginate as compared to hydrocolloid.

In this type of question, choices other than the correct answer may be partially correct, but there can only be one best answer. In Question 1, the key word is "most." Although alginate impression material is pleasant tasting, has a pleasing color, and is easy to mix, these factors do not account for using alginate impressions material for preliminary impression procedures. Hydrocolloid impression material is used for final impression procedures only and is not used to take preliminary working impressions. Thus, the most important reason can only be (C), ability of alginate to withstand the pouring of multiple models from a single impression.

Strategies for Answering One Best Answer—Single-Item Questions

- Remember that only one choice can be the correct answer.
- Read the question carefully to be sure that you understand what is being asked.
- Quickly read each choice for familiarity. (This important step is often not done by test takers.)
- Go back and consider each choice individually.
- If a choice is partially correct, tentatively consider it to be incorrect. (This step will help you lessen your choices and increase your odds of choosing the correct answer.)
- Consider the remaining choices and select the one you think is the answer. At this point, you may want to quickly scan the stem to be sure you understand the question and your answer.
- Fill in the appropriate circle on the answer sheet. (Even if you do not know the answer, you should use your best judgment and make a selection. You are scored on the number of correct answers, so do not leave any blanks.)

Strategies for Answering Negative Format Questions

- Remember that you are using reverse logic reasoning.
- Focus on words that are capitalized in the stem of the question.
- Consider each choice option individually. Note that the incorrect options of a negative format question are written in a positive form.
- Your circled answer is the option choice that is the exception or least correct.

Negative Format Question

This type of question is used to test the exception to a general rule or principle. These questions can be tricky, since they require a reverse logic of reasoning for the examinee.

DIRECTIONS (Question 3): Each of the items or incomplete statements in this section is followed by suggested answers or completions. Select the ONE lettered answer or completion that is the EXCEPTION or false statement.

3. All of the following statements apply to interdental brushes **EXCEPT**
   a. they are useful in removing interproximal plaque.
   b. they are used where there is a space between the teeth.
   c. they are useful even when it is possible to remove plaque with a toothbrush around healthy tissues.
   d. they are useful in exposed furcation areas.

Note that unlike the one best answer—single-item question style, the negative format question is asking you to select the one answer that is false or the exception. Carefully read each of the choices to determine the positive options first. Remember that positive choices can be safely eliminated, since you are being asked to select the choice that is false. This process of elimination is sometimes easier to think through and allows the correct choice—the exception—to stand out quickly. In this particular case, options (A), (B), and (D) are positive or true in reference to interdental brushes and are, therefore, incorrect answer choices. By eliminating these three positive options, only choice (C) remains. Choice (C) is the correct answer because it is the exception, or false statement. If plaque can be removed easily with a toothbrush and the tissue is healthy, an interdental brush is not necessary.

Matching Question

These questions are essentially matching questions that are always accompanied by the following general directions.

Strategies for Answering Matching Questions

- As with single-item questions, these questions have only one best answer.
- Carefully read through each option in Column B with every item question in the matching set before selecting your final answer.
- Refer to strategies under One Best Answer—Single-Item Questions for additional information.

DIRECTIONS (Questions 4 through 8): Match the items in Column A with their primary function in Column B.

Column A	Column B
4. spoon excavator	A. used to pack filling material
5. condenser	B. finishes or smooths restorations
6. scaler	C. effective in excavating soft caries
7. discoid–cleoid	D. used for removal of cement
8. ball burnisher	E. refines occlusal anatomy

A series of five questions usually is listed under Column A, with five answer choices under Column B. In this particular matching set, dental instruments are listed under Column A. Select the first item, question 4, spoon excavator, and systematically proceed to Column B, carefully reading all of the options and considering each choice individually. Continue this process with each item question 5, 6, 7, and 8. After reading each possible option in Column B, determine your correct choice on the answer sheet. As with single item questions, only one choice can be correct for a given question. For this reason, it is best to run through each question with all five option choices before entering your final answers. The correct answers for the matching set are as follows: 4 (C), 5 (A), 6 (D), 7 (E), 8 (B).

Complex Multiple-Choice—K-type Question

Complex Multiple-Choice—K-type Questions are no longer used on the DANB examination. A few sample questions are included in this text to promote critical thinking of related dental concepts. The reader may utilize and consider this information for general test-taking skills.

DIRECTIONS (Question 2): For each of the items in this section, ONE or MORE of the numbered options is correct. Choose answer
   A. if only 1, 2, and 3 are correct.
   B. if only 1 and 3 are correct.
   C. if only 2 and 4 are correct.
   D. if only 4 is correct.
   E. if all are correct.

Strategies for Answering Complex Multiple-Choice—K-Type Questions

- Carefully read and become familiar with the accompanying directions to this tricky question type.
- Read the stem to be certain that you know what is being asked.
- Read through each of the numbered choices. If you can determine whether any of the choices is true or false, you may find it helpful to place a "+" (true) or a "−" (false) next to the number.
- Focus on the numbered choices and your true/false notations, and use the following sequence to logically determine the correct answer.
  1. Note that in the answer code choices 1 and 3 are always both either true or false together. If you are sure that either one is incorrect, your answer must be (C) or (D).
  2. If you are sure that choice 2 and either choice 2 or 3 are incorrect, your answer must be (D).
  3. If you are sure that choices 2 and 4 are incorrect, your answer must be (B).
- Only one circle on the answer sheet must be filled in.

2. Some benefits of tray setups are
   1. they save time setting up.
   2. the dentist sets them up for the assistant.
   3. they eliminate delay in searching for instruments.
   4. they are used only in restorative procedures.
      A. 1,2,3
      B. 1,3
      C. 2,4
      D. 4
      E. All of the above

You first need to determine which choices are right and wrong and then which code corresponds to the correct numbers. In question 2, statements 1 and 3 are true, and therefore (B) is the correct answer.

➤ MULTIPLE-CHOICE TEST STRATEGIES

- Read the stem of the question carefully and completely before looking at the answers. Determine what the question is asking. Identify key words and then try to formulate the answer in your mind before looking at the answers.
- Read each answer carefully and determine whether it is an appropriate response to the question and gives as complete an answer as possible.
- Immediately eliminate any answers that are obviously incorrect and attempt to narrow the choices down to not more than two.
- When the choices have been narrowed as much as possible and the correct answer is still not clear, make an educated guess.

- Avoid selecting an answer because of complex choices or words and/or phrases that are unfamiliar to you.
- Watch for the words "not," "least," or "except" in the question.
- Look for the answer that best applies to the conditions presented in the question. An option may be partially true or may apply under certain conditions. Select the best answer that will generally apply under most conditions and specifically is applicable to the question. If several options might be true, but one option would incorporate all possibilities, that option should be the best answer.
- Be careful to mark the correct space on the answer sheet that relates to the item. Periodically review the answer sheet to make sure you have not inadvertently marked in the wrong space. After every ten questions, check to make sure you are on the same question in the test booklet as you are on the answer sheet.
- Listen carefully when instructions are given for marking the answer sheet. Do not assume it is just like others you may have used.
- If taking computerized format of the exam make sure you understand the program for marking correct answers.
- Avoid stray marks on the answer sheet if using the paper/pencil format.
- Never leave a question blank. There are no penalties for incorrect answers. By leaving a question blank, you may also increase your chances of marking the wrong space.
- Relax, put the test in perspective. The exam is only part of your education. Set yourself up for success by maintaining a positive attitude.

➤ TEST ANXIETY

It is impossible not to experience some anxiety when preparing to take the Dental Assisting Certification Examinations. Knowing the format of the board examinations will help reduce some of that anxiety. One method of reducing stress is to take practice tests to determine your individual strengths and weaknesses.

Adequately preparing for the Certification Board examinations will enable the candidate to think positively, reduce anxiety, and become confident in test-taking.

Try to get a good night's rest before the examination. Eating a light, well-balanced meal before the test will help you to stay alert. Maintain a positive attitude toward the test. Taking responsibility for your success is reflective in your preparation and attitude. Positive expectations bring positive results

Arrive at the test site early so you have time to relax. Practice relaxation exercises prior to the exam that will help alleviate anxiety. Stretching your neck, and shoulders may be helpful in relieving muscle tension. Come prepared with all of the materials that you will need, such as pencil, pen, wristwatch, identification, admission card, etc.

key concepts

Adequately preparing for the Certification Board Examinations will enable the candidate to think positively, reduce anxiety, and become confident in test taking.

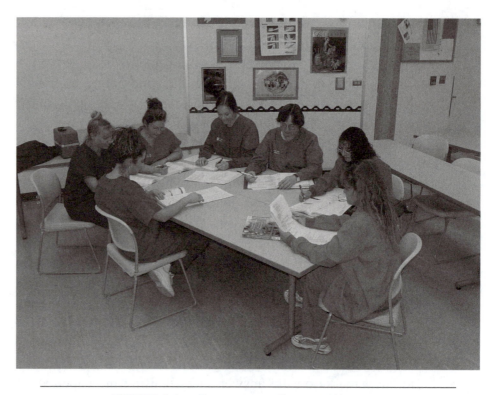

FIGURE 1-1.   Exam preparation—study group.

➤ EXAMINATION SCORING

Because there is no deduction for wrong answers, you should answer every question. The certification examination is not graded on a curve. Your test is scored in the following way.

1. **The Certified Dental Assisting Examination** consists of a total of 320 test questions; 120 questions are derived from general chairside assisting subject matter, 100 questions are derived from radiation health and safety, and 100 questions are derived from infection control. The test candidate must answer a minimum number of questions correctly in each of these three subject areas in order to successfully pass the certification examination. These minimum passing standards are calculated according to the number of correctly answered questions, which are individually scored according to item subject matter content and value of importance.

2. **The Specialty Certification Examination in Dental Practice Management Administrator** consists of a total of 275 test questions; 275 questions are specifically derived from that particular dental specialty.

3. **The Specialty Certification Examination in Orthodontics** consists of a total of 300 questions; 200 questions are derived specifically from that particular dental specialty and the remaining 100 questions are derived from infection control. The test candidate must answer a minimum number of questions based on each of

these sections correctly in order to successfully pass the specialty certification examinations.

The examination may be repeated if failed following guidelines established by the DANB. Examination results are released in writing and issued directly to the test candidate only. All test candidates who pass the certification examinations successfully will receive a certificate designating them as a Certified Dental Assistant or a credential certifying them in a particular dental assisting specialty.

➤ PHYSICAL CONDITIONS

The DANB is very concerned that all their examinations be administered under uniform conditions in the numerous centers that are used. All test candidates are advised to protect the integrity of their answer choices. If the test candidate feels that the testing site facilities are too crowded or arranged in such a manner that would make it difficult to protect the answers, the candidate should inform the testing-site test administrator immediately.

Except for a No. 2 pencil and eraser, you are not permitted to bring anything (books, notes, reference materials) into the test room. A calculator is permitted for the Dental Practice Management Specialty Examination only. All candidates are required to bring their assigned admission card on the day of the examination and appropriate identification. No questions concerning the content matter of the examination may be asked during the testing session. Furthermore, no visitors will be permitted during the examination session. Late comers may be admitted but will not be allowed to write beyond the allotted examination testing time period.

CHAPTER

2

Biomedical Sciences

contents

➤ Systems of the Body

➤ Cytology and Histology

➤ Microbiology

➤ Oral Pathology

➤ Diseases of the Periodontium

➤ Dental Caries

➤ Oral Pathologic Conditions

➤ Autoimmune Disorders

➤ Lesions Associated with Infectious Diseases

➤ Pharmacology

This chapter provides an overview of the major systems of the human body, their physiologic functions, and significance to dental health. A synopsis of the closely related biomedical sciences of microbiology, oral pathology, and pharmacology is also presented.

KEY TERMS

Artery	Lymphadenopathy
Articulation	Lymphocytes
Axial	Parasympathetic
Bone marrow	Platelets
Cranial nerves	Ptyalin
Detoxification	Respiration
Digestion	Saliva
Homeostasis	Sympathetic
Hormones	Vein

➤ SYSTEMS OF THE BODY (Table 2–1)

I. SKELETAL SYSTEM

A. Bone is a rigid form of connective tissue that contains cells in an intercellular matrix or ground substance

1. Three types of cells are associated with bone
   a. Osteoblasts
   b. Osteocytes
   c. Osteoclasts
2. Within bone is a substance known as **bone marrow** which produces
   a. Red blood cells
   b. White blood cells
   c. Platelets

B. The human skeleton consists of 206 bones and is divided into two parts: axial and appendicular

1. Axial skeleton is comprised of
   a. Skull
   b. Vertebral column
   c. Ribcage
2. Appendicular skeleton is comprised of bones associated with the body's appendages

TABLE 2–1   SYSTEMS OF THE BODY

1. Skeletal system	6. Respiratory system
2. Muscular system	7. Digestive system
3. Nervous system	8. Excretory system
4. Circulatory system	9. Endocrine system
5. Lymphatic system	10. Reproductive system

C. Bones are connected at joints or **articulations**; there are three types of joints
   1. Synarthrotic joints join bones in close contact and do not move, such as the sutures of the skull
   2. Amphiarthrotic joints have limited movement
   3. Diarthrotic joints are freely movable, such as the temporomandibular joint, joining the maxilla and mandible

II. MUSCULAR SYSTEM
A. Three types of muscle fibers
   1. Striated—voluntary in action and attached to the skeleton
   2. Smooth—involuntary not consciously controlled such as respiratory system
   3. Cardiac—specialized involuntary muscle found in heart

B. Muscle reflexes are actions causing an uncontrollable reaction
   1. Gagging
   2. Swallowing
   3. Coughing

III. NERVOUS SYSTEM
A. The two major segments of the nervous system include:
   1. Central nervous system—brain and spinal cord
   2. Peripheral nervous system—composed of all other nerves of the body
      a. Autonomic nervous system maintains bodily **homeostasis**
      b. **Sympathetic**
      c. **Parasympathetic**

B. Cranial nerves are 12 paired nerves that control major functions of the body including sight, smell, and taste (Table 2–2)

TABLE 2–2   CRANIAL NERVES

Cranial Nerves	Function
I Olfactory	Smell
II Optic	Sight
III Oculomotor	Movement of eyes
IV Trochlear	Movement of eyes
V Trigeminal	Chewing, conduction of sensation, and movement by the ophthalmic, maxillary, and mandibular nerves to the face
VI Abducens	Movement of eyes
VII Facial	Secretion of saliva, taste, facial expression
VIII Auditory (acoustic)	Hearing and balance
IX Glossopharyngeal	Taste, swallowing, secretion of saliva
X Vagus	Slowing of heart beat, increase in peristaltic movement
XI (Spinal) Accessory	Movement of shoulder and head
XII Hypoglossal	Movement of tongue, speech

Circulatory System

Heart
Blood vessels
Blood
Red blood cells—erythro-
cytes
White blood cells—leuko-
cytes
Platelets

IV. CIRCULATORY SYSTEM IS COMPRISED OF THE HEART, BLOOD VESSELS, AND BLOOD

A. Arteries carry blood away from the heart to all other parts of the body

1. Thick, elastic vessels that expand and contract as heart pumps blood
2. Pulse rate is the number of heart contractions during a given period of time
3. Systole occurs when heart contracts
4. Diastole occurs when heart is in a relaxed phase
5. Measurement of arterial pressure corresponds to body's blood pressure

B. Veins carry blood back to the heart

1. Veins are thinner than arteries.
2. Veins possess small valves that prevent blood from flowing backward.

C. Capillaries are the smallest blood vessels and appear in the greatest number; blood and cells exchange nutrients, oxygen, and waste products at the capillary level

D. Blood is composed of a liquid component called plasma and solid components that include:

1. **Red blood cells**—erythrocytes produced in bone marrow contain hemoglobin that transports oxygen to the cells.
2. **White blood cells**—leukocytes include lymphocytes used in body's defense mechanism.
3. **Platelets**—responsible for clotting process.

V. LYMPHATIC SYSTEM

A. Organs of the lymphatic system include:

1. Lymph nodes—swelling is referred to as **lymphadenopathy**
2. Tonsils
3. Thymus
4. Spleen

B. Lymph nodes filter the lymph fluid and produce **lymphocytes and monocytes which destroy microorganisms in the body** (Figure 2–1)

Lymphatic System Organs

Lymph nodes
Tonsils
Thymus
Spleen

VI. RESPIRATORY SYSTEM

A. Respiration is the process by which the oxygen required by each cell for the production of energy is introduced into the bloodstream, and carbon dioxide, a waste product of cellular activity is removed

B. Transfer of gases occurs in the lungs where thin-walled capillaries are in close proximity to the alveoli, or air sacs of the lungs

VII. DIGESTIVE SYSTEM

A. The alimentary canal is composed of five organs: the oral cavity, esophagus, stomach, and small and large intestines

Digestive System Organs

Oral cavity
Esophagus
Stomach
Small intestine
Large intestine

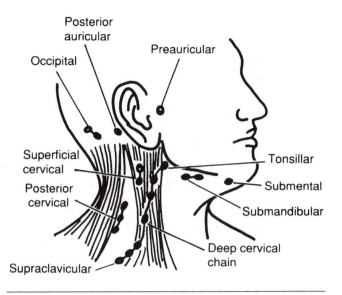

FIGURE 2–1. Lymph nodes of the head and neck.

B. Saliva contains the digestive enzyme **ptyalin, which begins the breakdown of starches in the mouth**
  1. Teeth function to break up food
     a. Incisors used for biting
     b. Canines used for tearing
     c. Premolars and molars used for crushing and grinding
  2. Food bolus is lubricated by saliva produced in the salivary glands
     a. Parotid salivary gland
     b. Submandibular salivary gland
     c. Sublingual salivary gland

C. The liver is an adjunct organ of the digestive system and is involved in the formation of bile
  1. Liver **detoxifies** harmful chemicals that enter the body
  2. Local anesthetics are broken down in the liver

VIII. EXCRETORY SYSTEM

A. Excretory system functions to remove waste products from the body, supporting the maintenance of homeostasis

B. Organs of the excretory system include skin, lungs, intestines, and urinary tract

IX. ENDOCRINE SYSTEM

A. Endocrine system is responsible for secreting hormones, which regulate metabolic functions of the body

B. Organs of the endocrine system include the pituitary, thyroid, parathyroid, pineal, adrenal glands, pancreas, and the gonads

C. Pancreas secretes insulin which promotes the use of glucose in cells and thereby decreases blood glucose concentration.
  1. Insulin is essential for the maintenance of normal levels of blood glucose

Glands of the
Endocrine System

Pituitary gland
Thyroid gland
Parathyroid gland
Pineal gland
Adrenal gland
Pancreas
Gonads

2. Increase in the level of blood glucose is known as diabetes mellitus caused by inadequate supply of insulin in the body

D. Estrogen and progesterone can exert harmful gingival effects during pregnancy

E. Imbalance in release of thyroid hormone can affect the development and eruption rate of teeth

X. REPRODUCTIVE SYSTEM

A. Humans reproduce sexually; fertilization is the fusion of the nuclei of the female egg and the male sperm

B. Development of the face of the embryo begins between the third and twelfth week of pregnancy
   1. Teeth begin to develop at about the sixth week of gestation
   2. Tetracycline taken during the last trimester of pregnancy can cause discoloration of the teeth of the infant

C. Pregnant women are to be draped with a lead-lined apron and exposed to the least amount of radiation possible if radiographs are necessary; the fetus is most vulnerable during the first trimester

XI. CYTOLOGY AND HISTOLOGY

A. Cytology is the study of cells
   1. Cell is the basic unit of life
   2. Cells have three major functions
      a. Respiration
      b. Reproduction
      c. Locomotion
   3. Mitosis is the process of cell division, the result of mitosis is the production of a second cell that contains identical genetic materials (chromosomes) to the original cell
   4. Chromosomes are filamentous structures in the cell nucleus and contain genes
   5. Genes are the basic units of heredity and are capable of self-replication
   6. DNA deoxyribonucleic acid is the basic carrier of genetic information in the cells

B. Histology is the microscopic study of the structure of tissues
   1. Four basic types of tissues
      a. Epithelial—acts as covering or lining of body system
      b. Connective—supports or binds body organs together
      c. Muscle—specialized tissue coordinates motor/sensory functions
      d. Nervous—specialized tissue coordinates motor/sensory functions
   2. Individual cells that form an organ or specialized tissue are related and perform specialized functions

XII. MICROBIOLOGY

A. Microbiology is the study of biologic microorganisms which can only be seen with the aid of a microscope

B. Three major classifications of microorganisms
1. Viruses—pathologic conditions include:
a. Herpes simplex
b. Hepatitis
c. HIV—Human immunodeficiency virus
2. Fungi—include yeasts and molds
a. Intraoral diseases
b. Candidiasis or thrush
3. Bacteria—dental caries and periodontal disease

C. Tuberculosis is caused by a resistant bacteria tubercle bacilli

XIII. ORAL PATHOLOGY

A. Oral pathology is a recognized dental specialty concerned with the disease processes of the oral cavity
1. Developmental disturbances—cleft lip or palate
2. Infectious diseases—herpes simplex
3. Nutritional deficiencies—chelitis
4. Cancer-related abnormal growths

B. Specific pathology tests include:
1. Biopsy is performed by surgically removing a small specimen of abnormal tissue for further diagnosis (Figure 2–2)
a. Benign—nonmalignant lesion
b. Malignant—cancerous lesion

C. Exfoliative cytology is a nonsurgical procedure performed by scraping the surface of the lesion with a moistened wooden tongue blade and transferring the specimen to a prepared slide for definitive study under the microscope

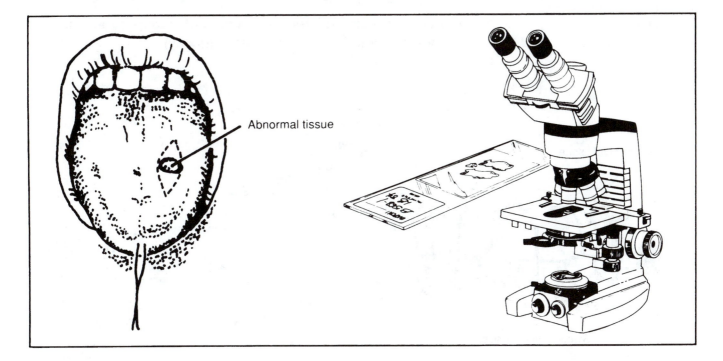

Abnormal tissue

FIGURE 2–2. Pathology tests.

Diseases of the Periodontium

Gingivitis
Periodontitis
ANUG—acute necrotizing ulcerative gingivitis
Pregnancy gingivitis

Dental Caries

Disease involving the demineralization of enamel
Affects the dentin and cementum
Caused by acid-producing bacteria and refined carbohydrates

XIV. DISEASES OF THE PERIODONTIUM

A. Gingivitis is a disease of the periodontium involving inflammation of the gums (Figure 2–3)
1. Characterized by red, edematous, tender gingiva that may bleed easily
2. Prevented by eliminating plaque through daily brushing, flossing, and use of interdental cleaning devices

B. Periodontal disease that affects the alveolar bone is called periodontitis
1. Untreated gingivitis may turn into periodontitis
2. Characterized by inflamed gingival tissues that bleed easily
   a. Periodontal pocket formation
   b. Loss of alveolar bone
   c. Furcation involvement in multirooted teeth
   d. Gingival recession
   e. Tooth mobility
   f. Exudate upon probing in advanced cases
3. Treatment of periodontal disease involves debridement, scaling, rootplaning and surgical procedures

C. Acute necrotizing ulcerative gingivitis (ANUG) also known as trench mouth or Vincent's infection is characterized by ulcerated gingiva and a gray pseudomembrane

D. Pregnancy gingivitis is characterized by enlarged swollen gingival tissues that bleed easily
1. Pregnancy tumor is called pyogenic granuloma
2. Hormonal changes contribute to enlargement of gingival tissues

XV. DENTAL CARIES

A. Acid-producing bacteria in the form of plaque is responsible for the promotion of dental caries (decay)

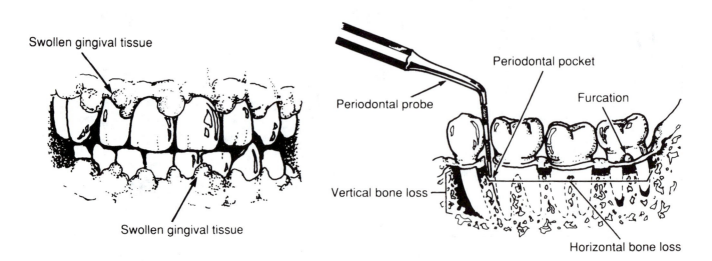

Swollen gingival tissue

Swollen gingival tissue

Periodontal pocket

Periodontal probe

Furcation

Vertical bone loss

Horizontal bone loss

FIGURE 2–3. Gingival inflammation and periodontal involvement.

B. Dental caries is responsible for the destruction and demineralization process that affects the enamel, dentin, and cementum

C. Untreated dental caries (decay) can lead to pulpal disease
1. Pulpitis
2. Pulp stones or denticles
3. Hyperemia
4. Periapical abscesses

XVI. ORAL PATHOLOGIC CONDITIONS
A. Developmental pathologic conditions that affect the teeth
1. Anodontia—a lack of development of the teeth
2. Supernumerary teeth—excess number of teeth
3. Microdontia—teeth that are small in size
4. Macrodontia—teeth that are large in size
5. Amelogenesis imperfecta—anomalies during formation of enamel
6. Dentinogenesis imperfecta—anomalies during the formation of dentin
7. Dilaceration—formation of roots with sharp bends
8. Fusion—two teeth partially or completely join or fuse resulting in a single large tooth
9. Gemination—attempted division of the tooth bud, two incomplete teeth develop
10. Concrescence—after root formation cementum or two teeth is joined

B. Most common developmental pathologic conditions include a cleft of either the lip or the palate

C. Developmental pathologic conditions that affect the tongue
1. Cleft tongue—fusion of the two halves of the tongue is incomplete
2. Fissured tongue—abnormal number of grooves or fissures on dorsal side of the tongue
3. Geographic tongue—papillae on the tongue lose their surface epithelium
4. Hairy tongue—hypertrophy, overgrowth of the filiform papillae
5. Glossitis—inflammatory condition of the tongue
6. Nutritional vitamin B deficiency—pellagra, tongue appears bright red and has a burning sensation

D. Common oral pathologic conditions that may be left untreated
1. Fordyce granules—elevated sebaceous glands
2. Tori—bony protrusions appearing on the palate or mandible
3. Abrasion—pathologic wearing away of tooth structure
4. Attrition—normal wearing away of the functional biting surfaces or the teeth by mastication, bruxism
5. Erosion—loss of tooth structure through a chemical process
   a. Associated with nutritional eating disorders
   b. Anorexia nervosa
   c. Bulimia
   d. Decalcification of enamel surfaces

Developmental Pathologic Conditions

Anodontia—lack of teeth
Supernumerary teeth—excess number of teeth
Microdontia—small teeth
Macrodontia—large teeth
Gemination—division of tooth bud
Fusion—two teeth fuse
Dilaceration—sharp bend in roots
Amelogensis imperfecta—affects enamel
Dentinogensis imperfecta—affects dentin
Cleft lip/palate

Lesions of the Tongue

Cleft tongue
Fissured tongue
Geographic tongue
Hairy tongue
Glossitis

Common Oral Pathologic Conditions

Fordyce granules—elevated sebaceous glands
Tori—bony growth on palate or floor of mouth
Abrasion—pathologic wear of tooth
Attrition—wear of biting surfaces
Erosion—loss of tooth by chemical process

E. Tumors are areas of swollen tissue often found in the oral cavity (the word tumor does not imply a cancerous or carcinogenic lesion)
1. Benign tumors of the oral cavity
    a. Papilloma
    b. Pigmented nevi
    c. Fibroma
    d. Hemangioma
    e. Pyogenic granuloma
    f. Leukoplakia
2. Malignant tumors of the oral cavity, head, and neck region
    a. Basal cell carcinoma
    b. Squamous cell carcinoma—epidermoid
    c. Melanoma

XVII. **AUTOIMMUNE DISORDERS**
A. Recurrent aphthous ulcers are commonly referred to as canker sores
1. Lesion looks ulcerated and is painful
2. Lesion occurs anywhere in the oral cavity—lip, cheek, tongue, floor of mouth

B. Etiology is unknown indicative of an altered autoimmune response of the oral epithelium or physical trauma

C. Immunity is the property of a host to resist specific infections
1. Acquired immunity can be produced by an injection of antibodies of one person into another (e.g., immunization)
2. Acquired immunity can be produced by the formation of antibodies in a person as a result of previous exposure to a microorganism

D. Host may be born with natural antibodies against specific microorganisms, which is termed natural immunity

XVIII. **LESIONS ASSOCIATED WITH INFECTIOUS DISEASES**
A. Herpes simplex, commonly known as herpes or cold sores, is a contagious viral infection characterized by blister-like lesions that usually appear on the lips

B. Varicella, commonly known as chickenpox, is highly contagious; lesions may occur intraorally

C. Mumps, or parotitis, involves unilateral or bilateral swelling of the parotid and other salivary glands; mumps is contagious

D. Moniliasis is an infection caused by a fungus, *Candida albicans;* candidiasis (thrush) can occur in infants and debilitated persons, frequently associated with patients who have HIV

E. Acquired immunodeficiency syndrome (AIDS) is an infectious disease that attacks the human immune system
1. Oral lesions include herpes simplex, Kaposi's sarcoma
2. Candidiasis, hairy leukoplakia of the tongue, ANUG

Lesions Associated with Infectious Disease

Herpes simplex—herpes, viral
Varicella—chicken pox, viral
Mumps—swelling of parotid gland
Moniliasis—candidiasis or thrush, fungal
Kaposi's sarcoma—AIDS
Oral chancre—primary stage syphilis

F. Syphilis is a highly contagious disease transmitted through sexual contact
   1. Primary stage—chancres soft tissues of oral cavity
   2. Secondary state—mucous patches appear on the tongue
   3. Teritary syphilis—necrotized gumma oral lesion

XIX. PHARMACOLOGY

A. Pharmacology is the scientific body of knowledge concerned with the properties of drugs and the interactions of chemical compounds within living systems

B. Commonly used drugs in dentistry include:
   1. **Antibiotics**—aid in defense mechanisms of the body by inhibiting growth or destroying invading bacteria
   2. **Sedatives and hypnotics**—central nervous depressants produce a calming effect for anxious dental patients
   3. **Non-narcotic analgesics**—assist in alleviating mild to moderate pain after dental procedures

C. Prescription is a written order directing a pharmacist to dispense a certain drug with specific instructions to a patient (Figure 2–4)
   1. Dentist is only oral health-team member to legally prescribe drugs
   2. All prescriptions must be written in ink
   3. Duplicate copy of the prescription must be recorded in the patient's dental chart for legal purposes

D. Methods of drug administration
   1. Orally is the most common method
   2. Inhalation method has a quick onset
   3. Topically—on the surface
   4. Sublingually—under the tongue
   5. Injection—forcing of a fluid into a vessel or cavity
   6. Intravenous—into the vein
   7. Intramuscular—into the muscle

Methods of Drug Administration	
Topical	Intramuscular
Oral	Intradermal
Sublingual	Subcutaneous
Inhalation	Parenteral
Injection	Rectally
Intravenous	

```
DEA #
              John Smith, D.D.S.
              Address
              Telephone

Name:                          Date:
Address:                       Age:

    RX
        Tetracycline USP, 250 mg
        Dispense: 30 capsules
        Signature: Take 2 stat and 1 q.i.d. subsequently


Refill _____        _____ D.D.S.
```

FIGURE 2–4.   Sample prescription order.

8. Intradermal—just breaking the skin surface
9. Subcutaneous—under the skin deeper than intradermal
10. Parenteral—any route other than the alimentary canal
11. Rectally—pertaining to the rectum

E. Proper handling of drugs—ordering and inventory

1. Careful records must be kept of all prescription drugs ordered for the dental office
2. Inventory is required on a periodic basis to monitor and control the potential abuse of prescription drugs
3. Narcotic drugs must be stored in a locked cabinet

F. Storage of prescription drugs

1. Drugs should be stored according to the manufacturer's directions
2. Nitroglycerin has a short shelf life if stored in the office emergency kit must be replaced every six months
3. Check expiration dates; discard appropriately

G. Telephone procedures for inquiries related to prescriptions dictate that the dental auxiliary is not authorized by law to phone in a prescription for a patient

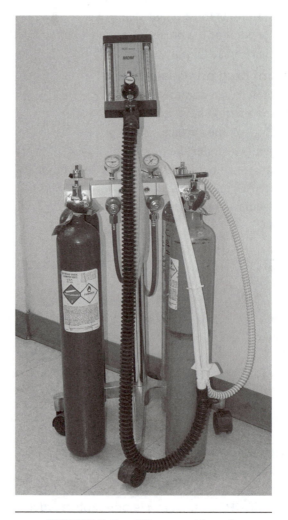

FIGURE 2–5. Nitrous oxide unit.

H. Categories of medications

1. **Analgesics**—administered to relieve mild to moderate pain include aspirin
2. **Local Anesthesia**—administered by injection
   a. Lidocaine (Xylocaine)—local anesthetic
   b. Mepivacaine (Carbocaine)—local anesthetic
   c. some local anesthetics contain Epinephrine
3. **Anesthetics**—may be general, as in surgical procedures
   a. inhalation method of administration
   b. intravenous method of administration
4. **Nitrous Oxide**—inhalation method of administration, beneficial for patients who are anxious or apprehensive (Figure 2–5)
5. **Antibiotics**—destroy or inhibit the growth of bacteria
   a. Penicillin
   b. Amoxicillin
6. **Antifungal Agents**—administered for treatment of fungal infections of the oral cavity, e.g., Nystatin
7. **Antihistamines**—effective in cases of severe allergic reaction
8. **Central Nervous System Depressants**—barbiturates which are sedative hypnotics principally used to induce sleep, reduce anxiety, and alleviate convulsions
9. **Central Nervous System Stimulants**—rarely prescribed by dentists, e.g., amphetamines affect the cerebral cortex and cause restlessness and alertness
10. **Narcotics**—potent analgesics (pain-relieving drugs), e.g., codeine, meperidine (Demerol), and morphine

Categories of Medications

Analgesics
Anesthetics
  General
  Local
  Nitrous oxide
Antibiotics
Antifungal
Antihistamine
CNS depressants
CNS stimulants
Narcotics

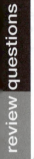

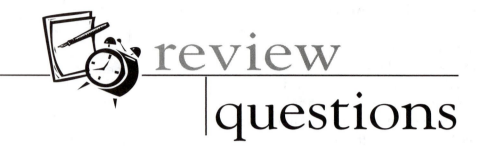

review questions

DIRECTIONS Each of the questions or incomplete statements below is followed by suggested answers or completions. Select the **one answer** that is best in each case.

1. A written direction to a pharmacist to prepare a drug is called a (an)
   A. invoice.
   B. contract.
   C. prescription.
   D. order blank.

2. The cells that produce bone are
   A. osteoblasts.
   B. ameloblasts.
   C. odontoblasts.
   D. fibroblasts.

3. Joints that do not move are called
   A. hinge joints.
   B. gliding joints.
   C. temporomandibular.
   D. synarthrotic joints.

4. The abbreviation q4h means
   A. every four days.
   B. every four hours.
   C. take before meals.
   D. as needed.

5. The cranial nerve controlling tongue movements is the
   A. obiculoris oris.
   B. trigeminal.
   C. vagus.
   D. hypoglossal.

6. HIV/AIDS is a disease of the
   A. endocrine system.
   B. digestive system.
   C. immune system.
   D. reproductive system.

7. The function of the epiglottis is to
   A. control the tidal volume of air.
   B. support the pituarity gland.
   C. regulate the CO_2 and O_2 ratio of inspired air.
   D. prevent liquids and solids from entering the respiratory system.

8. Inspiration is caused by
   A. a decrease in size of alveoli.
   B. expansion of the pleural cavity.
   C. relaxation of the diaphragm.
   D. contraction of the chest.

9. The function of hemoglobin is to
   A. carry nutrients.
   B. fight infection.
   C. transport oxygen.
   D. stimulate endocrine glands.

10. Blood platelets are necessary in
    A. allergic reactions.
    B. antigen-antibody reactions.
    C. CO_2 elimination.
    D. blood clotting.

11. The number of chambers in the human heart is
   A. one.
   B. two.
   C. three.
   D. four.

12. The arterial pulse indicates the
   A. blood pressure.
   B. number of times the heart is contracting.
   C. temperature of the blood.
   D. cardiac output.

13. The diastolic blood pressure is the pressure exerted by blood on the walls of the
   A. arteries when the heart is at rest.
   B. veins when the heart pumps.
   C. arteries when the heart pumps.
   D. veins when the heart is at rest.

14. Lymph nodes function to
   A. transport nutrients.
   B. produce plasma.
   C. produce lymphocytes.
   D. store leukocytes.

15. Digestion begins in the
   A. large intestine.
   B. oral cavity.
   C. small intestine.
   D. stomach.

16. Absorption of most nutrients occurs in the
   A. small intestine.
   B. stomach.
   C. large intestine.
   D. esophagus.

17. Congenital refers to
   A. a condition existing at birth.
   B. a condition that worsens during aging.
   C. diseases of the teeth.
   D. diseases of the parents.

18. Endocrine glands affect the body by chemical mediators called
   A. lymphnodes.
   B. hormones.
   C. impulses.
   D. genes.

19. The hormone released during times of dental stress is
   A. epinephrine.
   B. estrogen.
   C. ptyalin.
   D. progesterone.

20. The liver functions to
   1. metabolize fat
   2. detoxify harmful substances
   3. manufacture bile
   4. manufacture genes

   A. 1, 2
   B. 1, 3
   C. 3 only
   D. 1, 2, 3
   E. All of the above

answers & rationales

1.

C. A prescription is a written direction to a pharmacist to prepare a drug. A prescription includes the following information: doctor's name, address, and telephone number; patient's name, address, and age; date; drug name and dosage; quantity of the drug; directions for use; and doctor's signature and DEA (narcotic registration number).

2.

A. Cells involved in the production, maintenance, and resorption of bone are osteoblasts, osteocytes, and osteoclasts, respectively. Osteoblasts produce a prebony matrix that is then calcified. They then become osteocytes, which are responsible for maintaining bone. Osteoclasts cause the resorption of bone by secreting enzymes that dissolve the bony matrix.

3.

D. A joint is the junction of bones. The types of joints are synarthroses, which do not move, such as those found in the skull; amphiarthroses, those with limited movements, such as those between vertebrae; and diarthroses, the most mobile, such as the temporomandibular joint. A suture is a type of joint that does not move.

4.

B. Some common Latin abbreviations are **q4h** (every 4 hours), **qid** (4 times a day), **prn** (as needed), and **ac** (before meals).

5.

D. The hypoglossal nerve controls tongue movement.

6.

C. AIDS is a disease of the immune system. The acquired immunodeficiency syndrome (AIDS) is a fatal condition with a variety of symptoms that affect the entire body, including the oral cavity. AIDS is caused by the human immunodeficiency virus (HIV).

7.

D. The epiglottis prevents solids and liquids from entering the respiratory system by closing the entrance of the larynx.

8.

B. Inspiration is caused by expansion of the pleural cavity. This is accomplished by the contraction of the diaphragm and the intercostal muscles., causing the alveoli to expand and create a vacuum. Expiration is the reverse of inspiration.

9.

C. Hemoglobin is a red pigment in red blood cells that transports oxygen to cells and helps remove carbon dioxide from cells.

10.

D. The sequence in blood clotting is:
a. broken blood vessels → breakdown of platelets → platelet factors

b. platelet factors + antihemophilic factor → thromboplastin

c. prothrombin + thromboplastin → thrombin

d. fibrinogen + thrombin → fibrin

11.

D. The heart is composed of four chambers: two atria and two ventricles. The atria have thinner walls and are collecting chambers, receiving blood from the body and the lungs. The ventricles contain more muscle tissue and pump the blood to the lungs and the body.

12.

B. The arterial pulse normally indicates the number of times the heart is contracting. Other characteristics of the pulse, such as rhythm and strength, are indications of the cardiac condition.

13.

A. Diastolic blood pressure is the pressure exerted by blood on the walls of arteries when the heart is at rest. Systolic blood pressure is the pressure exerted on the walls of arteries when the heart contracts. In healthy young adults, the average blood pressure is 120/80.

14.

C. Lymph nodes function to filter lymph and to produce lymphocytes and antibodies.

15.

B. Digestion begins in the oral cavity. The enzyme ptyalin, contained in the saliva, begins the digestion of starch and lubricates the food bolus. The tongue pushes the food bolus downward into the esophagus, which connects the oral cavity to the stomach.

16.

A. Absorption of most nutrients occurs in the small intestine. The surface area of the small intestine is greatly enlarged by the number of surface projections, called villi.

17.

A. Congenital refers to a condition that exists at or before birth. Some common congenital defects of the oral cavity are missing teeth, alteration in the enamel an dentin, cleft palate, and many facial defects.

18.

B. Endocrine glands produce chemical mediators called hormones. Hormones are proteins distributed via the circulatory system.

19.

A. Epinephrine is produced by the medullary portion of the adrenal glands during times of stress. It increases the heart rate, constricts most arterioles, and increases the blood pressure. The effects of epinephrine are similar to the effects of the sympathetic division of the autonomic nervous system.

20.

D. The liver functions to metabolize fats, carbohydrates, and proteins, to produce bile and blood proteins, to detoxify harmful substances, to produce body heat, and to store vitamins.

Dental Anatomy

contents

➤ Anatomic Landmarks of the Skull

➤ Soft Tissue Landmarks of the Oral Cavity

➤ Salivary Glands

➤ The Tongue

➤ The Major Muscles

➤ Oral Embryology

➤ Tooth Morphology

➤ Occlusion

➤ The Periodontium

This chapter presents the basic hard and soft tissue anatomic landmarks of the skull and oral cavity. A synopsis of the development of teeth and individual tooth morphology descriptions of the permanent and primary dentition are presented.

KEY TERMS

Calcification	Molar
Canine	Occlusion
Cranium	Periodontium
Exfoliate	Premolar
Gingiva	Succedaneous
Incisors	Trigeminal nerve
Mandible	Temporomandibular joint
Maxilla	

Cranial Bones

Frontal (1)
Parietal (2)
Temporal (2)
Occipital (1)
Sphenoid (1)
Ethmoid (1)

Facial Bones

Zygomatic (2)
Maxilla (2)
Nasal (2)
Lacrimal (2)
Palatine (2)
Vomer (1)
Inferior concha (2)
Mandible (1)

Salivary Glands and Ducts

Parotid gland—Stenson's duct
Submandibular gland—Wharton's duct
Sublingual gland—ducts of Rivinus

I. ANATOMIC LANDMARKS OF THE SKULL (Figures 3–1 and 3–2)

A. The **cranium** (skull) is composed of 22 bones
   1. There are 8 bones in the cranium (Table 3–1)
   2. The face contains 14 bones (Table 3–2)

B. Upper jaw or **maxilla** contains the upper teeth

C. Lower jaw or **mandible** contains the lower teeth (Figures 3–3 and 3–4)

D. The range of motion of the mandible is defined by the **temporomandibular joint**

II. SOFT TISSUE LANDMARKS OF THE ORAL CAVITY (Figures 3–5 and 3–6)

A. Oral cavity bound by lips and cheeks externally

B. Oral cavity proper bound by alveolar arches, teeth, fauces, hard and soft palate, and tongue

C. Roof of mouth is formed by the palate
   1. Hard palate separates the oral and nasal cavities
   2. Soft palate is muscular and functions in speech

III. SALIVARY GLANDS

A. The oral cavity contains three major paired salivary glands
   1. Parotid glands
      a. Located in front of and just below each ear
      b. Secretes saliva through Stensen's duct
   2. Submandibular glands
      a. Located on the inner surface at the angle of the mandible
      b. Secretes saliva through Wharton's duct
   3. Sublingual glands located under the tongue
      a. Secretes saliva through major sublingual duct (Bartholin's)
      b. Secretes saliva through ducts of Rivinus

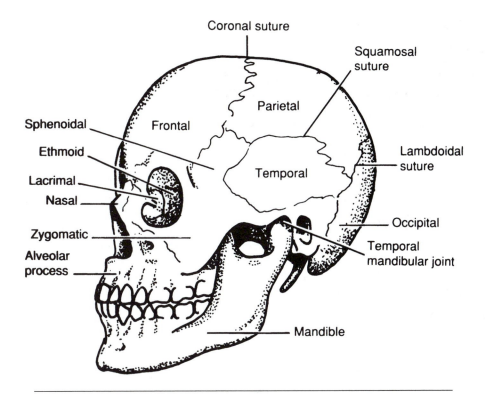

FIGURE 3–1.   Bones of the cranium (lateral view).

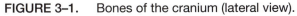

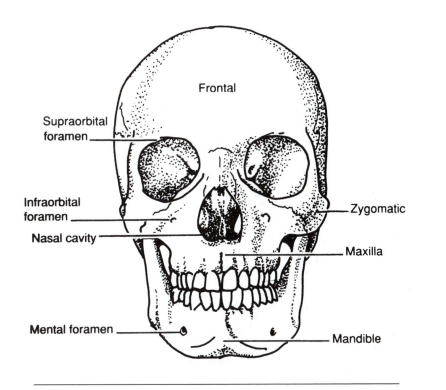

FIGURE 3–2.   Bones of the face (frontal).

TABLE 3–1	BONES OF THE CRANIUM
Bones	**Anatomic Landmarks**
Frontal (1)	Superior anterior and roof of the skull; contains the frontal sinuses
Parietal (2)	Superior medial sides and roof of the skull
Temporal (2)	Medial sides of the skull; contains the middle ear, inner ear
Occipital (1)	Posterior base of the skull; posterior wall and posterior floor of cranial cavity
Sphenoid (1)	Anterior base of skull behind orbits
Ethmoid (1)	Part of nose, orbits, and floor of cranial cavity

TABLE 3–2	BONES OF THE FACE
Bones	**Anatomic Landmarks**
Zygomatic (2)	Forms the prominence of the cheeks, lateral wall, and floor of the orbit
Maxilla (2)	Helps form the boundaries of the roof of the mouth, provides support for teeth of the upper arch; contains the maxillary sinus
Nasal (2)	Bridge of the nose
Lacrimal (2)	Anterior part of medial wall of the orbit
Palatine (2)	Floor of nasal cavity, floor of the orbit
Vomer (1)	Posterior and inferior portion of nasal septum
Inferior concha (2)	Lateral wall of nasal cavity
Mandible (1)	Consists of body, ramus, and angle; forms lower jaw and provides support for teeth; range of motion is defined by temporomandibular joint

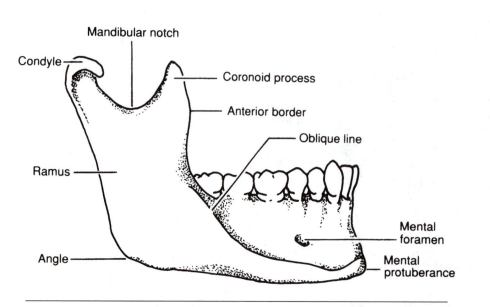

FIGURE 3–3. External aspect of the mandible.

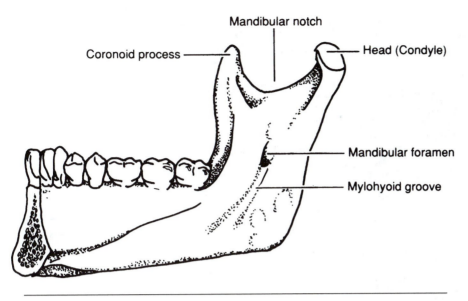

FIGURE 3–4.   Internal aspect of the mandible.

B. Saliva is the liquid medium that distributes basic digestive enzymes

C. Saliva lubricates the oral tissues and functions to maintain balance of the oral bacteria

IV. THE TONGUE FUNCTIONS IN SPEECH AND MASTICATION AND IS THE MAJOR ORGAN OF TASTE CONTAINING THE TASTE BUDS (Figure 3–7)

V. THE MAJOR MUSCLES

A. Muscles of mastication function in the movement of the mandible

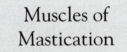

Muscles of Mastication

Temporal
Internal (medial) pterygoid
External (lateral) pterygoid
Masseter

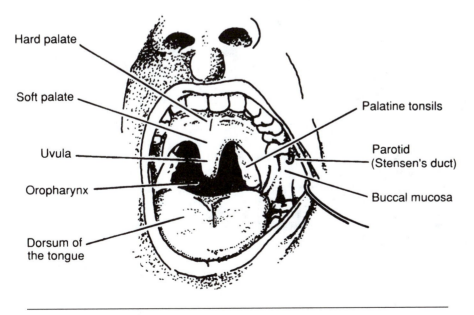

FIGURE 3–5.   Soft tissue landmarks of the oral cavity.

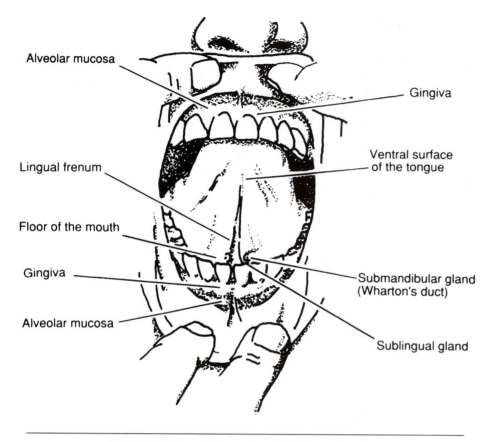

Alveolar mucosa

Gingiva

Lingual frenum

Ventral surface of the tongue

Floor of the mouth

Gingiva

Submandibular gland (Wharton's duct)

Alveolar mucosa

Sublingual gland

FIGURE 3–6. Salivary glands in the oral cavity.

B. Each side of the face has four major muscles (Figure 3–8)
1. Temporal muscle
2. Internal (medial) pterygoid muscle
3. External (lateral) pterygoid muscle
4. Masseter muscle

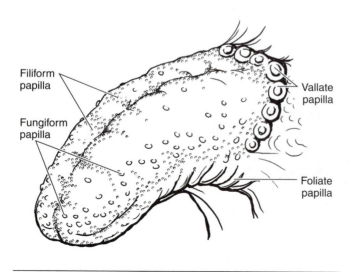

Filiform papilla

Vallate papilla

Fungiform papilla

Foliate papilla

FIGURE 3–7. Dorsal surface of the tongue—taste buds.

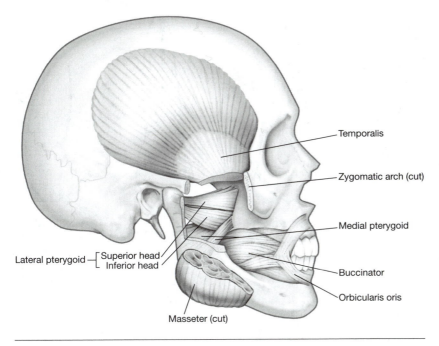

Temporalis

Zygomatic arch (cut)

Medial pterygoid

Lateral pterygoid — Superior head
　　　　　　　　　Inferior head

Buccinator

Orbicularis oris

Masseter (cut)

FIGURE 3–8.　Muscles of mastication. (From Brian, J. & Cooper, M. (2002). *Complete Review of Dental Hygiene* (p. 62). Upper Saddle River, NJ: Prentice Hall. Reprinted with permission.)

C. All muscles of mastication are innervated by the **trigeminal nerve** (fifth cranial nerve)

D. Muscles of facial expression

VI. ORAL EMBRYOLOGY

A. Teeth begin developing at approximately 6 weeks in utero

B. Formation of tooth buds leads to development of primary and **succedaneous** teeth

C. Tooth buds mature and develop distinct shapes during the apposition and **calcification** stage

D. Primary teeth begin to **exfoliate** at approximately 6 years of age when succedaneous teeth begin to erupt

VII. TOOTH MORPHOLOGY (Figure 3–9)

A. Shape of each tooth is determined by its specific function

1. **Incisors** are designed to cut food
2. **Canines** are designed to cut or tear food
3. **Premolars** are designed for tearing and grinding food
4. **Molars** are designed for grinding food

B. Permanent dentition

1. Eight incisors
   a. Central incisors erupt age 7 to 8
   b. Lateral incisors erupt age 8 to 9
2. Four canines
   a. Maxillary canines erupt age 11 to 12
   b. Mandibular canines erupt age 9 to 10

Muscles of Facial Expression

Mentalis
Orbicularis oris
Buccinator
Zygomaticus

Types of Teeth

Incisors
Canines
Premolars
Molars

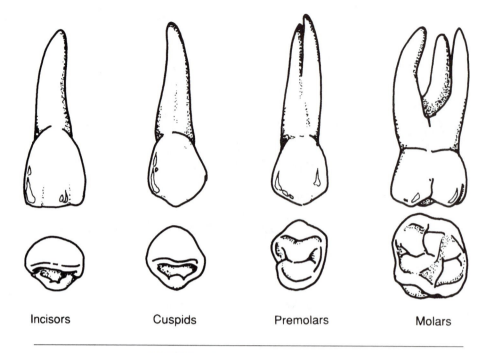

Incisors   Cuspids   Premolars   Molars

FIGURE 3–9. Tooth morphology.

   3. Eight premolars
      a. Maxillary first premolars erupt age 10 to 11
      b. Maxillary second premolars erupt age 10 to 12
      c. Mandibular first premolars erupt age 10 to 12
      d. Mandibular second premolars erupt age 11 to 12
   4. Twelve molars
      a. Maxillary first molars erupt age 6
      b. Maxillary second molars erupt age 12
      c. Maxillary third molars erupt age 17 to 21
      d. Mandibular first molars erupt age 6
      e. Mandibular second molars erupt age 12
      f. Mandibular third molars erupt age 17 to 21

C. Primary dentition
   1. Eight primary incisors
      a. Maxillary central incisors erupt 7 ½ months
      b. Maxillary lateral incisors erupt 9 months
      c. Mandibular central incisors erupt 6 months
      d. Mandibular lateral incisors erupt 7 months
   2. Four primary canines
      a. Maxillary canines erupt 18 months
      b. Mandibular canines erupt 16 months
   3. Eight primary molars
      a. Maxillary first molar erupt 14 months
      b. Maxillary second molar erupt 24 months
      c. Mandibular first molar erupt 12 months
      d. Mandibular second molar erupt 20 months
      e. There are no premolars in the primary dentition

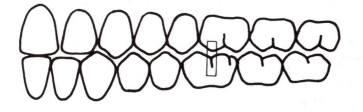

FIGURE 3–10. Class I neutrocclusion. Classification based on relationship of the first permanent molars.

VIII. OCCLUSION (Figures 3–10 and 3–11)

A. **Occlusion** is the study of how the masticatory system operates; includes placement of teeth in the arch, articulation, and the action of the supporting joints and muscles; normal or ideal occlusion has a molar relationship similar to Class I with no malpositioned teeth

　　1. Angles classification of malocclusion (Table 3–3)

　　　　a. Class I malocclusion—Neutrocclusion

　　　　b. Class II malocclusion—Distocclusion

　　　　c. Class III malocclusion—Mesiocclusion

TABLE 3–3　OCCLUSAL RELATIONSHIPS AND CLASSIFICATION OF MALOCCLUSION

Occlusal Relation	Molar Relationship	Canine Relationship	Facial Profile
Normal (Ideal) Occlusion	Mesiobuccal cusp of maxillary first permanent molar occludes with buccal groove of mandibular first permanent molar.	Maxillary permanent canine occludes with distal half of mandibular canine and mesial half of mandibular first premolar.	Orthognathic
Class I Malocclusion— Neutrocclusion	Mesiobuccal cusp of maxillary first permanent molar occludes with buccal groove of mandibular first permanent molar. Malposition of individual teeth or groups of teeth	Malposition of individual teeth or groups of teeth	Orthognathic
Class II Malocclusion— Distocclusion Class II—Division 1 Mandible is retruded and all maxillary incisors are protruded Class II—Division 2 Mandible is retruded and one or more maxillary incisors are retruded	Buccal groove of mandibular first permanent molar is distal to mesiobuccal cusp of maxillary first permanent molar (by at least width of premolar).	Distal surface of mandibular canine is distal to mesial surface of maxillary canine (by at least width of premolar).	Retrognathic
Class III Malocclusion— Mesiocclusion	Buccal groove of mandibular first permanent molar is mesial to mesiobuccal cusp of maxillary first permanent molar (by at least width of premolar).	Distal surface of mandibular canine is mesial to mesial surface of maxillary canine (by at least width of a premolar).	Prognathic

2. Malocclusion can lead to unbalanced distribution of the forces of mastication and to severe dental problems

B. Centric occlusion—when teeth are at maximum intercuspation

C. Overjet—horizontal distance between upper and lower anterior teeth

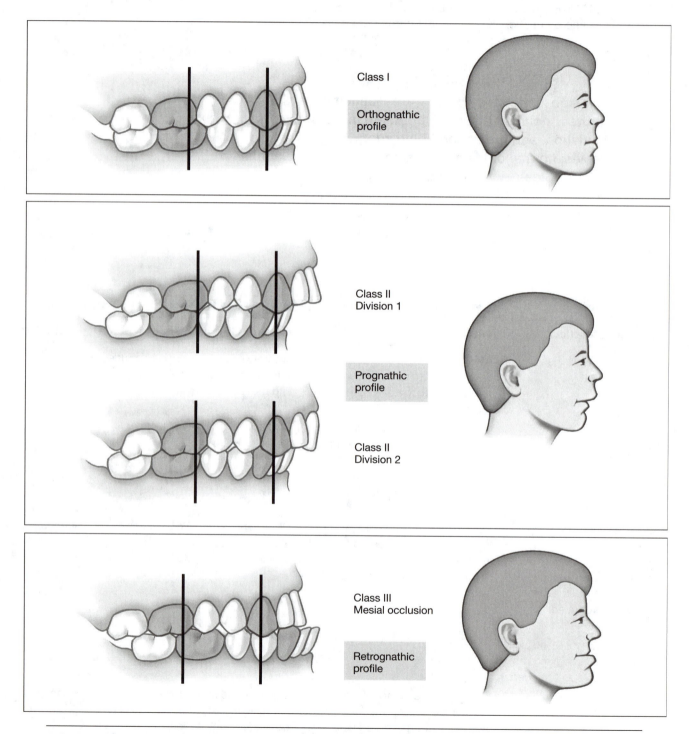

FIGURE 3–11. Occlusal relationships. Class I (top); Class II, division 1 (middle top); Class II, division 2 (middle bottom); Class III (bottom). (From Brian, J. & Cooper, M. (2002). *Complete Review of Dental Hygiene* (p. 311). Upper Saddle River, NJ: Prentice Hall. Reprinted with permission.)

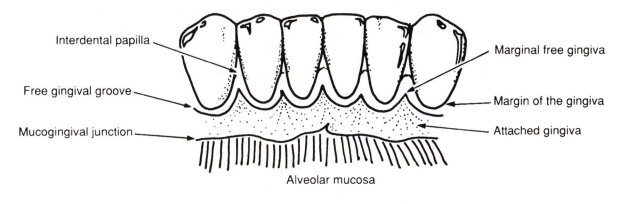

FIGURE 3–12.   Periodontium: gingival tissues.

D. **Overbite**—vertical distance between upper and lower anterior teeth

E. **Crossbite**—maxillary teeth are positioned lingual to the mandibular teeth may occur unilaterally or bilaterally

F. **Openbite**—abnormal vertical space between mandibular and maxillary teeth, most frequent in anteriors

IX. THE PERIODONTIUM (Figures 3–12 and 3–13)

A. The **periodontium** consists of those tissues that support tooth function
   1. Gingiva
   2. Alveolar bone
   3. Periodontal ligament
   4. Cementum

> **Periodontium Tissues**
>
> Gingiva
> Alveolar bone
> Periodontal ligament
> Cementum

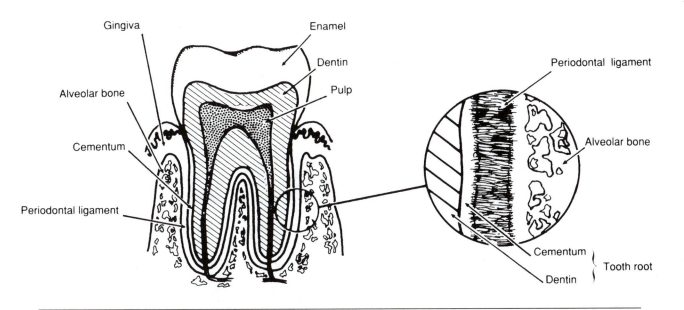

FIGURE 3–13.   Periodontium: individual tooth and structures.

B. Healthy gingival sulcus when measured with a periodontal probe will have a measurement depth of 3mm or less

C. Periodontal ligament encloses each tooth and serves to connect the alveolar bone to the cementum

D. Cementum is a hard tissue that covers the root surface of each tooth

E. Alveolar bone (process) provides a bony socket and support for each tooth in the dentition

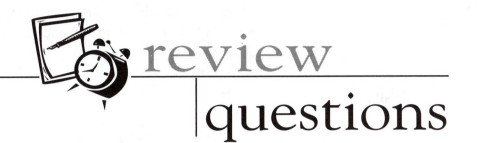

questions

review questions

DIRECTIONS Each of the questions or incomplete statements below is followed by suggested answers or completions. Select the **one answer** that is best in each case.

---

1. The type of bone supporting the teeth is called
   A. cortical bone.
   B. periodontal bone.
   C. alveolar bone.
   D. attached bone.

2. Which is the most prominent bone making up the skeletal structure of the cheek?
   A. vomer
   B. mandibular
   C. ethmoid
   D. zygomatic

3. The maxillary tuberosity is located
   A. anterior to the maxillary sinus.
   B. posterior to the maxillary third molar.
   C. lateral to the masseter muscle.
   D. posterior to the mandibular third molar.

4. Which tooth is most often located under the maxillary sinus?
   A. maxillary central incisor
   B. maxillary lateral incisor
   C. maxillary cuspid
   D. maxillary first molar

5. The muscle surrounding the opening of the mouth is the
   A. buccinator.
   B. obicularis oris.
   C. medial pterygoid.
   D. masseter.

6. The muscles of mastication are innervated by the
   A. facial nerve.
   B. trigeminal nerve.
   C. lingual nerve.
   D. cranial nerve.

7. The blood vessels supporting the head with blood are the
   A. common carotid arteries.
   B. brachial arteries.
   C. pulmonary arteries.
   D. radial arteries.

8. A frenum is a fold of mucous membrane. Frena are located
   1. in the maxillary labial vestibule.
   2. at the junction of the hard and soft palate.
   3. in the mandibular labial vestibule.
   4. at the retromolar ridge.
      A. 1 only
      B. 1 and 2
      C. 2 and 3
      D. 1 and 3
      E. 4 only

9. The periodontium consists of the
   1. gingiva.
   2. alveolar process.
   3. cementum.
   4. periodontal ligament.

A. 1 only
B. 1 and 2
C. 2 and 4
D. 1, 2, and 3
E. All of the above

10. The major salivary glands include all of the following EXCEPT the
    A. sublingual gland.
    B. parotid gland.
    C. submandibular gland.
    D. pituarity gland.

11. The parotid gland is located
    A. under the tongue.
    B. along the inferior border of the mandible.
    C. below and in front of the ear.
    D. adjacent to the thyroid gland.

12. Which part of the tooth forms first?
    A. crown
    B. root
    C. pulp
    D. dentin

13. Each developmental lobe on molars is represented by a
    A. fissure.
    B. cusp.
    C. marginal ridge.
    D. groove.

14. Angle's classification of malocclusion is based on the
    A. shape of the maxilla.
    B. relationship between the first molars and the orbit of the eye.
    C. relationship between the maxillary and mandibular first molars.
    D. number of teeth in the mandible.

15. The gingival sulcus
    A. lies between the free and attached gingiva.
    B. is on the labial surface of anterior teeth.
    C. is on the alveolar mucosa.
    D. lies between the tooth and the internal surface of the free gingiva.

16. Exfoliation is the
    A. internal absorption of succedaneous teeth.
    B. removal of permanent teeth.
    C. shedding of primary teeth.
    D. technique used to perform a biopsy.

17. The surface of the tooth facing the midline of the mouth is the
    A. mesial.
    B. distal.
    C. lingual.
    D. incisal.

18. How many root canals does the maxillary first premolar have?
    A. one
    B. two
    C. three
    D. four

19. The cusp of Carabelli is sometimes found on what tooth?
    A. maxillary first premolar
    B. maxillary second premolar
    C. maxillary first molar
    D. mandibular second molar

20. The surface of the anterior teeth facing the lips is the
    A. buccal.
    B. facial/labial.
    C. palatal.
    D. occlusal.

✓answers & rationales

1.

C. The bone that supports the teeth is called the alveolar bone. Other names for alveolar bone are cancellous or medullary bone. Fibers of the periodontal membrane are inserted into the part of the alveolar bone known as the lamina dura.

2.

D. The zygomatic bone is the most prominent facial bone and is also called the cheekbone.

3.

B. The maxillary tuberosity is a bony structure located posterior to the maxillary third molar. It is the distal extension of the alveolar ridge.

4.

D. The teeth most often found below the maxillary sinus are the maxillary second premolars, first molars, and second molars. Inflammation of the maxillary sinus (sinusitis) can result when these teeth are percussed.

5.

B. The orbicularis oris is the muscle that surrounds the mouth. It functions to close the lips, press the lips against the teeth, and protrude the lips.

6.

B. The muscles of mastication are all innervated by the mandibular branch of the trigeminal nerve.

7.

A. The blood vessels that supply blood to the head are the right and left common carotid arteries.

8.

D. Frena are located between the upper mucous membrane and the gingiva located between the upper central incisors, the lower mucous membrane and the gingiva located between the lower central incisors, and the mucous membrane on the floor of the mouth and the underside of the tongue. If the lingual frenum is short, the tongue is limited in movement, and the patient is known as tongue-tied.

9.

E. The periodontium consists of the periodontal membrane, the alveolar bone, the gingiva, and cementum.

10.

D. The sublingual, parotid, and submandibular glands are the major salivary glands.

11.

C. The parotid glands, are located below and in front of the ears. The glands become enlarged when a person has the mumps.

12.

A. The first part of the tooth to be formed is the crown. It is not until the enamel and dentin have reached the future cementoenamel junction that root formation begins.

13.

B. The developmental lobe on molars is represented by a cusp. The mandibular first molar is formed by the fusion of five developmental lobes, whereas the mandibular second molar is formed by the fusion of four developmental lobes.

14.

C. Angle's Classification of malocclusion is based on the relationship between the maxillary and mandibular first molars. When the teeth are in normal (ideal) occlusion the mesiobuccal cusp of the maxillary first molar fits in the buccal groove of the mandibular first molar. Deviations of occlusion classification include: the mandibular molars are one cusp distal to their normal position (Class II distoclusion) and the mandibular molars are one cusp mesial to their normal position (Class III mesioclusion). Class I malocclusion is similar to normal (ideal) occlusion in molar relationship with malpositioned individual or groups of teeth.

15.

D. The gingival sulcus is bordered by the tooth, the internal surface of the free gingiva, the gingival attachment, and the oral cavity.

16.

C. Exfoliation is the shedding of primary teeth. This is an active process that occurs between the ages of 6 and 12 years and is caused by the resorption of the roots of the primary teeth.

17.

A. The surface of the tooth that faces the midline is the mesial surface. The surface that is the farthest from the midline is the distal surface.

18.

B. The maxillary first premolar usually has two roots, buccal and palatal, as well as two root canals.

19.

C. The cusp of Carabelli is the fifth cusp sometimes present on the palatal surface of the mesiolingual cusp of the maxillary first molar. The cusp is non-functional.

20.

B. Anteriorly, the surface of the teeth facing the lips is the labial surface. Posteriorly, the surface of the teeth facing the cheek is the buccal surface. The surface of the upper teeth facing the palate is the palatal surface. The surface of the lower teeth facing the tongue is the lingual surface.

4

Preventive Dentistry

contents

➤ Soft Deposits

➤ Hard Deposits

➤ Toothbrushes and Brushing Techniques

➤ Dental Floss and Flossing Technique

➤ Oral Physiotherapy Devices

➤ Fluorides

➤ Dental Sealants

➤ Nutrition and Diet Analysis

➤ Plaque-Control Programs

This chapter addresses the basic skills and concepts for preventing dental disease, including oral physiotherapy techniques, plaque etiology, nutritional counseling, plaque control programs, fluoride therapy, and the application of dental sealants.

KEY TERMS

Bacterial plaque	Materia alba
Calculus	Mottled enamel
Demineralize	Nutrients
Disclosing agent	Plaque control
Extrinsic stain	Recall (recare)
Fluoride	Sealants
Interproximal brush	Sulcus
Intrinsic stain	

I. SOFT DEPOSITS

A. Bacterial Plaque

1. Soft, sticky, dense, gelatinous layer of bacteria
2. Adheres to teeth and gingival tissues
3. Removed by proper toothbrushing methods, flossing, and use of interdental devices

B. Stages of Plaque Formation

1. Early stage—pellicle, colorless
2. Later stages—thick, whitish appearance
   a. Composed of organized bacteria
   b. Held together in sticky matrix
   c. Plaque maturation occurs within 12 to 24 hours
      1) Carbohydrates and sucrose in diet increase plaque production
      2) Plaque produces irritants (acids)
      3) **Demineralization** of tooth enamel leads to dental caries.
      4) Plaque irritants create gingival inflammation

C. Materia Alba

1. Loosely attached thick soft deposit
2. Removed by vigorous rinsing or water irrigating device
3. Associated with poor oral hygiene

D. Dental Stains

1. **Extrinsic stains** coat outer surfaces of teeth
2. Removed by coronal polishing techniques
3. Range in color
   a. Yellow stain caused by poor oral hygiene
   b. Brown stain caused by food pigments, chlorhexidine rinse
   c. Green stain caused by remnants of Nasmyth's membrane
   d. Black line stain caused by chromogenic bacteria
   e. Tobacco stain caused by tar/tobacco by products
   f. Orange and red stain caused by chromogenic bacteria

4. **Intrinsic stains**
   a. Systemic disorders may cause intrinsic stains
   b. Medications—tetracycline cause intrinsic gray color to enamel
   c. **Mottled enamel**—intrinsic stain; color range yellowish-brown or white spots—pitted
   d. Dental fluorosis caused by excess 2 parts per million (ppm) fluoride in the drinking water during mineralization of tooth formation
   e. Cannot be removed by coronal polishing techniques

II. HARD DEPOSITS
A. Calculus
1. Hard mineralized mass of bacterial plaque
2. Removed by hand instruments such as scalers, curettes
3. Removed by powered instruments sonics, ultrasonics

B. Formation of Calculus
1. Supragingival calculus above the gingival margin
2. Subgingival calculus below the gingival margin

III. TOOTHBRUSHES AND BRUSHING TECHNIQUES
A. Bass technique (Figure 4–1)
1. Emphasizes sulcular brushing
2. Bristles of toothbrush placed at 45-degree angle

B. Charters technique most effective when interdental spaces are open
C. Modified Stillman technique incorporates a rolling stroke and vibratory stroke; bristles do not enter **sulcus**
D. Rolling stroke technique—bristles on gingival tissues blanch then roll onto occlusal surfaces

> ### Toothbrushing Methods
>
> Bass technique
> Charters technique
> Modified Stillman technique
> Rolling stroke technique

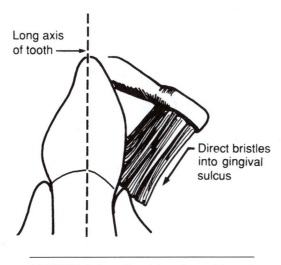

Long axis of tooth

Direct bristles into gingival sulcus

FIGURE 4–1. Toothbrush positioned for sulcular brushing.

Oral Physiotherapy Devices

Disclosing agents
Interproximal brushes
Toothpaste—dentifrice
Cosmetic/therapeutic
　mouthrinses
Perio aids/piks
Rubber gingival tip stimulator
Floss holder
Wooden interdental wedge
Floss threader
Water irrigation devices
Partial clasp brush
Denture brush—immersion
　agent

IV. DENTAL FLOSS AND FLOSSING TECHNIQUE (Figure 4-2)

A. Dental floss is used to remove interproximal plaque
B. Specialty floss for fixed bridgework, implants

V. ORAL PHYSIOTHERAPY DEVICES

A. Toothpaste and dentifrices provide therapeutic benefits
　1. Fluorides reduce incidence of dental caries
　2. Desensitizing agents reduce tooth sensitivity
B. Mouthrinses may be classified as cosmetic and therapeutic
C. **Disclosing agents** identify plaque by coloring the deposit
D. **Interproximal brushes** are used to remove plaque in furcations and large interdental spaces
E. Perio aids are used to cleanse under the gingival margin
F. Rubber tip stimulators are useful in reshaping the gingiva after periodontal surgery
G. Wooden interdental cleaner for wide interproximal areas
H. Floss holder is beneficial for patients who have difficulty manipulating the dental floss
I. Floss threader is used to thread floss under and between pontic of fixed bridges and orthodontic wires
J. Water irrigator removes loose food debris around teeth; useful for orthodontic patients

VI. FLUORIDES

A. **Fluoride** is a mineral nutrient
　1. Applied topically
　2. Administered systemically through water supply
　3. Vitamin supplements
B. Fluoridation of water supply effective at 1 part per million (ppm); May be adjusted for warmer or colder climates
C. Topical fluoride agents and characteristics (Table 4-1)
　1. Sodium fluoride available in 2% aqueous solution
　2. Acidulated phosphate fluoride

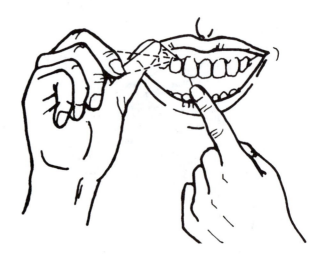

FIGURE 4-2.　Flossing technique.

TABLE 4-1	COMPARISON OF TOPICAL FLUORIDE CHARACTERISTICS	
Fluoride Agent	Advantages	Disadvantages
Sodium fluoride (NaF) 2%	Does not stain teeth Stable solution when stored in polyethylene bottle Less objectionable taste Gingival irritation does not occur	Success of treatment dependent on series of several appointments
Acidulated phosphate fluoride (APF) 1.23% NaF with 0.1 M orthophosphoric acid	Does not stain teeth Stable when stored in polyethylene bottle Pleasant taste may be flavored Requires single application	Can irritate inflamed ginvigal tissues May cause etching effects on resin restoration or porcelain
Stannous fluoride (SnF$_2$) 0.4%	Available in liquid solution May be incorporated in dentifrice for caries control Brush-on gel form available for patient home use	Taste is objectionable May cause staining of teeth Short shelf-life May be irritating to inflamed gingival tissues

   3. Stannous fluoride used as desensitizing agent 0.4% gel
   4. Neutral sodium used for porcelain and composite restorations.

D. Fluoride toxicity is a potential danger if the correct dosage of fluoride is not administered

VII. DENTAL SEALANTS
A. Pit and fissure **sealants** are applied to the occlusal surfaces of caries-free teeth
B. Dental sealants are etched with phosphoric acid prior to application of the resin

VIII. NUTRITION AND DIET ANALYSIS
A. Nutrition is a combination of basic food elements and **nutrients**
B. The six key nutrient groups (Table 4–2)
   1. Proteins
   2. Carbohydrates
   3. Fats
   4. Minerals
   5. Vitamins
   6. Water
C. Five food groups provide the sources for a balanced diet (Figure 4–3)
   1. Milk, yogurt, and cheese group
   2. Meat, poultry, fish group
   3. Fruit group

USDA Recommended 5 Food Groups

Bread, cereal, pasta, rice group (6–11 daily servings)
Vegetable group (3–5 daily servings)
Fruit Group (2–4 daily servings)
Milk, yogurt, cheese group (2–3 daily servings)
Meat, poultry, fish, eggs, nuts, dried beans (2–3 daily servings)

TABLE 4–2   KEY NUTRIENTS

Nutrient	Functions	Sources	Deficiency
Proteins	Build and maintain body tissues; help body carry on normal processes	Meat, poultry, fish, milk, cheese, eggs, plants (soybean)	Kwashiorkor, marasmus
Carbohydrates	Supply energy	Sugars, syrups, cereals, grains, bread, jam and jelly, pasta, crackers, pretzels, dried fruits	None specifically, but excessive intake can lead to dental caries
Fats	Provide insulation and support for internal body organs	Oils, butter, egg yolks, nuts, meats	None, but excessive fat intake can lead to coronary disease
Minerals	Assist in the formation and maintenance of body structures and metabolism	Milk, meat, fish, nuts, whole grains, shellfish	Bone deformities, muscle tremors, anemia
Water	Essential for maintaining normal body processes and stable body temperature	Drinking water and other liquids	Dehydration, shock, death
Vitamins **Fat soluble**			
A	Assists in proper maintenance of epithelial cells, plays role in vision	Fish, liver, oils, vegetables, yellow fruits	Night blindness, severe drying of skin
D	Builds and maintains bones and teeth, regulates calcium and phosphorus metabolism	Milk, fish, eggs, liver, butter, sunshine	Rickets, poor tooth development
E	Essential for normal reproduction	Wheat germ, vegetable oil, green vegetables	Unknown
K	Contributes to normal blood clotting	Green vegetables, cabbage, cauliflower, soybean oil	Defective clotting
Water soluble			
C	Aids in resisting infections, healing, and maintaining a healthy gingiva, strengthens blood vessels	Citrus, fruits, brocolli, parsley, green vegetables, melons, tomatoes, berries	Scurvy
B_1 (thiamine)	Helps normal body function growth, assists in carbohydrate metabolism	Yeast, wheat germ, whole grains, pork, liver	Growth retardation, nerve disorders, beriberi
B_2	Contributes to normal function of body cells	Fish, eggs, whole grains, liver, meat, greens	Glossitis, cheilosis, dermatitis
B_6	Contributes to normal function of body cells	Meat, liver, vegetables, whole grain cereals	Anemia, skin lesions
B_{12}	Contributes to blood regeneration	Liver, milk, cheese	Pernicious anemia, neurologic disturbances
Niacin	Helps other cells use nutrients	Yeast, eggs, milk, green vegetables	Pellagra
Pantothenic acid	Assists in proper metabolism	Yeast, liver, kidney, eggs	Lack of proper metabolism
Folacin (folic acid)	Contributes to normal function of cells	Plant foods, greens, liver	Unknown
Biotin	Helps body use proteins, carbohydrates, and fats	Kidney, liver	Epithelial sensitivity, muscular pains

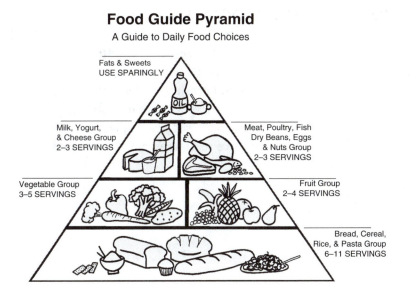

Food Guide Pyramid

A Guide to Daily Food Choices

FIGURE 4–3. Food guide pyramid. (From Brian, J. & Cooper, M. (2002). *Complete Review of Dental Hygiene* (p. 145). Upper Saddle River, NJ: Prentice Hall. Reprinted with permission.)

4. Vegetable group
5. Bread, cereal, pasta, and rice group

D. Snack foods that aid in the maintenance of good oral health

1. Fresh fruits and vegetables
2. Cheese, eggs
3. Nuts, lunch meats
4. Potato chips, popcorn
5. Milk, plain yogurt
6. Sugar-free soft drinks, unsweetened fruit juices

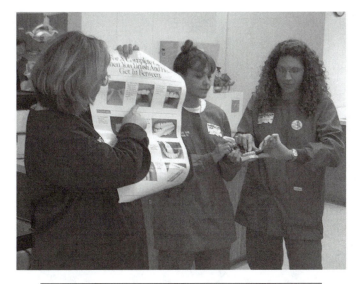

FIGURE 4–4. Plaque control programs.

IX. PLAQUE CONTROL PROGRAMS (Figure 4–4)
A. Individualized plaque control programs assist to motivate the dental patient towards improved oral health
B. Sample plaque control program
   1. Visit #1—Basic instruction brushing, interdental devices, awareness
   2. Visit #2—Review, reinforce, reevaluate instructions
   3. Visit #3—Diet history review, suggest changes
   4. Visit #4—Provide positive reinforcement, set-up **recall** (recare appointment)

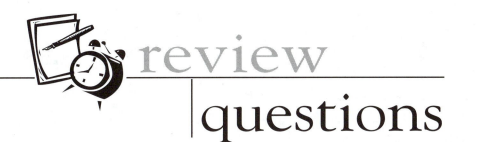

review questions

DIRECTIONS Each of the questions or incomplete statements below is followed by suggested answers or completions. Select the **one answer** that is best in each case.

1. What oral hygiene device should the auxiliary recommend to patients who have a fixed partial bridge?
   A. partial clasp brush
   B. denture brush
   C. mouth rinse
   D. bridge cleaners

2. What is considered to be the primary cause of dental disease?
   A. sugar
   B. plaque
   C. saliva
   D. materia alba

3. The first step in the formation of plaque is
   A. acquired pellicle.
   B. materia alba.
   C. food debris.
   D. bacterial colonization.

4. Which of the following nutrients has been found to be an overwhelming cause of the development of plaque and dental caries?
   A. proteins
   B. carbohydrates
   C. minerals
   D. vitamins

5. How often should a patient be recalled?
   A. every 9 months
   B. once a year
   C. whenever the patient decides

D. the time varies with the oral condition of the individual patients

6. Abrasion of the teeth may occur from using a
   A. hard bristle toothbrush.
   B. heavy waxed dental floss.
   C. medium bristle toothbrush.
   D. water irrigating devices.

7. How can one best motivate a patient when educating in the dental preventive philosophy?
   A. Present as much information as possible on the first visit.
   B. Provide a dental prophylaxis and fluoride treatment.
   C. Present information to the patient in a manner that will stimulate personal interest.
   D. Motivation is not a part of the auxiliary's responsibilities.

8. Periodontal disease may cause
   A. TMJ problems.
   B. dental caries.
   C. gums to recede.
   D. gums to become stippled.

9. Which of the following toothbrushing methods is the most effective method of removing plaque from the sulcus?
   A. rolling stroke method
   B. Bass method
   C. Charters method
   D. modified Stillman method

10. Disclosing agents identify
    A. plaque.
    B. carious lesions.
    C. calculus.
    D. gingival recession.

11. Which oral physiotherapy aid most appropriately is used to clean interdental areas when large interproximal spaces or open contacts exist?
    A. unwaxed dental floss
    B. perio aid
    C. denture brush
    D. interproximal brush

12. The sunshine vitamin is
    A. vitamin A.
    B. vitamin K.
    C. vitamin E.
    D. vitamin D.

13. A dilute sodium hypochlorite solution is recommended for cleaning
    A. partial dentures with metal clasps.
    B. full dentures.
    C. orthodontic bands.
    D. implants.

14. To be of maximum benefit to the teeth, the optimum fluoride concentration recommended is
    A. 1 ppm.
    B. 2 ppm.
    C. 100 ppm.
    D. 200 ppm.

15. Fluoride compounds most commonly used for topical application may include
    1. sodium fluoride.
    2. stannous fluoride.
    3. acidulated phosphate fluoride.
    4. prescription fluoride chewable tablets.
    A. 1, 3
    B. 2, 4
    C. 1, 2
    D. 1, 2, 3
    E. 4 only

16. Calculus (tartar) has the ability to irritate the gingival tissue because it is

    1. calcified.
    2. subgingival.
    3. covered with plaque.
    4. rough and irregular in texture.
    A. 1, 4
    B. 1, 3
    C. 2, 4
    D. 3 only
    E. All of the above

17. Foods that are high caries producers include
    1. nuts, cereals, grains.
    2. natural honey, raisins, syrup.
    3. fruits and vegetables.
    4. soft drinks, breath mints.
    A. 1, 2
    B. 1, 3
    C. 2, 4
    D. 4 only
    E. All of the above

18. Which of the following are considered detergent foods?
    1. apples, pears, water
    2. raisins, cheese, crackers
    3. lettuce, celery, carrots
    4. marshmallows, peanut butter, bananas
    A. 1 only
    B. 1, 3
    C. 2, 4
    D. 3 only
    E. 1, 2, 3, 4

19. The process of demineralization will occur with
    A. caries.
    B. calculus.
    C. green stain.
    D. yellow stain.

20. The best means of massage for the interdental papilla is the use of a
    A. perio aid.
    B. water irrigating device.
    C. balsa wood wedge.
    D. rubber tip stimulator.

✓answers & rationales

1.

D. A bridge cleaner is the best oral hygiene device to use for fixed partial bridgework. The bridge cleaner is threaded with dental floss, which can be inserted easily under the pontic of the fixed bridge.

2.

B. Bacterial plaque is the primary cause of dental disease. Microorganisms found in plaque produce harmful exotoxins that are acidogenic and lead to the demineralization of enamel and dental caries. Other mircroorganisms in bacterial plaque lead to the degeneration and irritation of the gingival tissues, causing gum disease.

3.

A. An acquired pellicle is the first step in plaque formation. Plaque requires 24 hours to mature, but a pellicle or film takes only minutes to form.

4.

B. Foods containing high levels of sugars are most responsible for producing caries. Carbohydrates have been found to be the most influential nutrient in causing caries. All carbohydrates are broken down to produce sugars, which interact with oral bacteria to form acids that can cause decay.

5.

D. The time between recall (recare) visits, examination, and oral prophylaxis varies according to the needs of the individual patient. Patients with a high caries index or those who are susceptible to periodontal disease are recalled more often than are patients who are less susceptible to oral disease. The usual time between recall (recare) visits is 6 months.

6.

A. In general, hard toothbrushes are not recommended because they can cause abrasion of the gingiva or enamel.

7.

C. Patient motivation is an important facet of the preventive dentistry philosophy. Patient education information should be presented in a manner that will stimulate the patient's specific dental health needs for best results and patient compliance.

8.

C. Peridontal disease may cause gums to recede. Recession of the gingival tissue is due to the apical migration of the junctional epithelium along the tooth surface, leading to apparent exposure of the root surface.

9.

B. The Bass technique is the most effective method of removing plaque from the sulcus because the bristles of the brush actually enter the sulcus. The Bass technique requires the bristles of a soft nylon brush to be placed at a 45-degree angle into the gingival sulcus. The brush is then rotated in small circular motions.

10.

A. Disclosing agents stain invisible plaque and, consequently, let the patient visualize this material.

Carious lesions, gingival recession, and calculus can be identified only through clinical examination.

11.

D. An interproximal brush is most effectively used when interdental spaces are sufficiently large. Dental floss is most effective in cases of tight contacts.

12.

D. Vitamin D, which is largely derived from sunshine, is instrumental in balancing the calcium and phosphorus ratio in the body. It is essential for bone and tooth formation.

13.

B. A dilute sodium hypochlorite solution, such as household bleach, is recommended for cleaning dentures. The technique is known as *immersion.* The solution is effective in removing light stains and dental plaque and serves as an antimicrobial agent for denture disinfection in the dental laboratory. Over-the-counter denture products, such as powders or tablets, also may be used. When cleaning partial dentures with metal framework, care must be taken to avoid tarnish or discoloration of the metals with certain immersion agents.

14.

A. The optimum amount of fluoride in drinking water is 1 ppm. Excessive amounts of fluoride (more than 2 ppm) may cause alteration in the calcification of enamel. The process of adding fluoride to the drinking water is called fluoridation.

15.

D. Fluoride compounds most commonly used for topical application include sodium fluoride, stannous fluoride, and acidulated phosphate fluoride gel.

16.

E. Calculus is a hardened or calcified material that can be removed only through mechanical means.

Calculus has a rough and irregular texture that tends to harbor plaque easily, leading to further gingival irritation and destruction. Calculus may be found subgingivally and supragingivally depending on location and severity of gingival disease.

17.

C. Foods that contain high levels of sugars are most responsible for producing caries. Such foods as honey and syrups are especially harmful because they stick or cling to the tooth surface for long periods of time, causing acid exposures. Soft drinks and candy mints also are recognized as high caries producers because of their high sucrose content.

18.

B. Detergent foods include fresh fruits and vegetables. Their textures actually help perform a cleansing action during the mastication process.

19.

A. The process of demineralization will occur with caries. When foods high in sucrose come in contact with bacterial plaque, they produce an acid that causes the tooth enamel to demineralize.

Sucrose + plaque = acid formation / dental decay (demineralization of enamel).

20.

D. Rubber tips are best used to stimulate interdental papilla. This process helps keratinize the gingiva and decrease inflammation. Balsawood wedges are used primarily to clean large interproximal tooth surfaces and secondarily to massage the papilla. Wedges are not as effective as rubber tips because they are stiffer and more difficult to manipulate.

5 Chairside Assisting

contents

➤ Zones of Operating Activity

➤ Charting—Universal Numbering System

➤ Periodontal Charting

➤ Dental Specialities

➤ Endodontics

➤ Oral and Maxillofacial Surgery

➤ Orthodontics

➤ Pedodontics

➤ Periodontics

➤ Prosthodontics

This chapter will provide a synopsis of general chairside dental assisting principles and procedures including four-handed sit-down dentistry concepts and dental charting techniques. An overview of the recognized dental specialties is presented with additional review material for chairside assisting in orthodontics.

KEY TERMS

Charting

Dental implant

Endodontics

Edentulous

Fixed prosthetic appliance

Malocclusion

Obturation

Oral and Maxillofacial Surgery

Orthodontics

Osseointegration

Pedodontics

Periodontics

Prosthodontics

Quadrant

Sedation

I. ZONES OF OPERATING ACTIVITY (Figure 5–1)
  A. Right-handed operator working zones are between 8 and 12 o'clock
  B. Dental assistant working zones are between 2 and 4 o'clock
  C. Transfer zone is where instrument transfers are made
    1. Instrument transfers are made at the patient's mouth or below the chin
    2. Transfer zone is between 4 and 8 o'clock
  D. Static zone contains less frequently used dental equipment
  E. Eye level of the dental assistant should be 6 inches above that of the operator

II. SEATING THE PATIENT
  A. Patient is seated and then reclined into a supine position
  B. Patient with respiratory and circulatory problems and in third trimester of pregnancy should be seated in an upright position
  C. Position the dental unit light for maximum illumination
    1. Direct beam of light upward for maxillary arch
    2. Direct beam of light downward for mandibular arch
  D. At the completion of a dental procedure slowly return the patient to an upright position, keep patient seated until equilibrium is regained

III. TRANSFERING OF INSTRUMENTS
  A. Instrument transfers require the use of Class I or Class II motions
    1. Class I motions involve the use of fingers for instrument transfer
    2. Class II motions involve fingers and wrist, for transfer of double-ended instruments
  B. Stages of instrument transfer
    1. Signal stage—operator makes a Class I motion moving the instrument out of the working field while maintaining the finger rest

---

Classification of Motion

Class I—Motion involves fingers as in instrument transfer

Class II—Motion involves fingers and wrist, for transfer of double-ended instruments

Class III—Motion involves use of fingers, wrist, and elbows

Class IV—Motion involves entire arm and shoulder as in reaching for overhead light.

Class V—Arm and torso movement as in turning, requires refocusing of the eyes

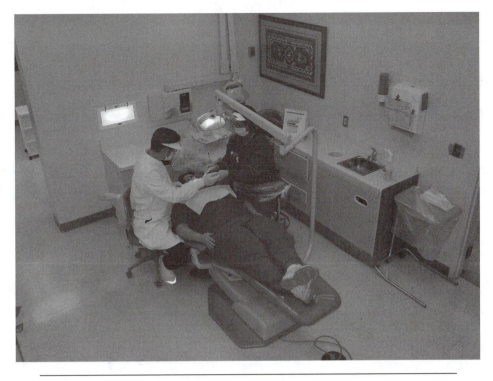

FIGURE 5–1. Zones of operating activity.

2. Pretransfer stage—assistant positions the instrument to be transferred parallel to the working instrument
3. Midtransfer stage—assistant holds the instrument to be transferred between the index finger and thumb and removes the instrument previously used from the operator's hand
4. Transfer stage—instrument to be transferred is placed in the proper position into the operator's hand
5. Transfer completion stage—assistant releases the transferred instrument and the operator returns to the operating field

C. Instrument grasps
1. Pen grasp used for hand instruments—explorers, spoon excavator
2. Chisels and hatchets are held in a palm-thumb grasp
3. Forceps and syringes are held in palm grasps

D. High-volume oral evacuation and retraction
1. Primary function is to provide a working field free of saliva and debris
2. Bacterial aerosol is decreased by use of the high-volume evacuator
3. Oral evacuator is positioned before the operator places the handpiece or mouth mirror
4. Oral evacuator may be used for retraction of the tongue and buccal mucosa

E. Tray setups decrease operatory prep time; instruments and materials routinely used 90% of the time are placed on preset trays

---

Stages of Instrument Transfer

Signal stage—operator moves instrument out of working field while maintaining a finger rest

Pre-transfer stage—assistant positions instrument

Mid-transfer stage—assistant removes instrument from operator and holds instrument to be transferred between thumb and index finger

Transfer stage—instrument to be transferred is placed in the operator's hand

Transfer completion—assistant releases transferred instrument and operator returns to operating field

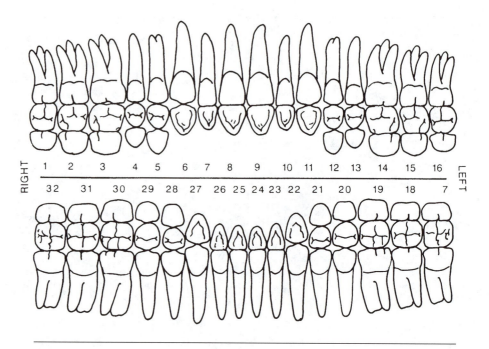

FIGURE 5–2. Adult dentition.

Tooth Charting Terminology

Mesial—tooth surfaces facing the mid-line
Distal—tooth surfaces facing away from the mid-line
Labial—anterior tooth surfaces facing the lips
Buccal—posterior tooth surfaces facing the cheeks
Lingual—tooth surfaces that face the tongue
Incisal—biting edges of anterior teeth
Occlusal—chewing surfaces of posterior teeth

IV. CHARTING

A. **Charting** is the process of recording the present condition of the hard and soft tissues in the oral cavity (Figure 5–2)
   1. Accurate charting is required for treatment planning and identification of accident victims
   2. Dental records may be used legally in a court of law involving malpractice suits
   3. Radiographs and study models are utilized to chart a patient's oral condition

B. **Location of each existing restoration and area of the oral cavity to be charted is identified in a standard manner**
   1. Mesial—tooth surfaces facing the midline
   2. Distal—tooth surfaces facing away from the midline
   3. Labial (facial)—tooth surfaces of anterior teeth facing the lips
   4. Buccal (facial)—tooth surfaces of posterior teeth facing the cheeks
   5. Lingual—tooth surfaces facing the tongue
   6. Incisal—biting edge of anterior teeth
   7. Occlusal—chewing surface of posterior teeth

C. **Symbols and abbreviations are used for dental charting**
   1. Blue-colored symbols designate existing treatment
   2. Red-colored symbols designate treatment to be performed

D. **Tooth identification systems**
   1. Universal system
      a. Identifies the adult dentition by numbers 1 through 32.
      b. Identifies the deciduous dentition by the letters A through T (Figure 5–3)

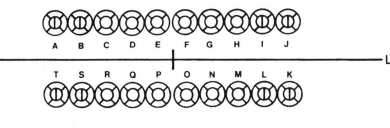

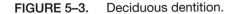

FIGURE 5–3. Deciduous dentition.

2. Palmer system
   a. Divides the mouth into **quadrants**; each quadrant is numbered 1 through 8
   b. Horizontal and vertical lines are used to indicate each individual quadrant
   c. Deciduous dentition is identified by letters A through E and is divided into quadrants
3. International system
   a. Divides the adult and deciduous teeth into quadrants
   b. Adult teeth in each quadrant are numbered 1 through 8
   c. Deciduous dentition is numbered 1 through 5

E. Periodontal charting records indications of periodontal disease activity.
   1. Six separate measurements are taken with a periodontal probe to record pocket depth (Figure 5–4)
   2. Charting symbols are used to indicate recession, mobility, root furcations, bleeding points, and suppuration
   3. Symbols are transferred directly onto the charting form to correspond with the exact location of the tooth

V. DENTAL SPECIALTIES

There are eight recognized dental specialties. The general dental practioner refers complex or difficult cases to the dental specialist for treatment

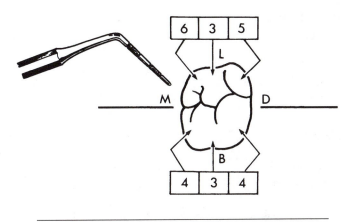

FIGURE 5–4. Periodontal charting.

Recognized Dental Specialties

1. Dental public health
2. Endodontics
3. Oral pathology
4. Oral and maxillofacial surgery
5. Orthodontics
6. Pedodontics
7. Periodontics
8. Prosthodontics

A. Dental public health

1. Public health dentistry includes community, municipal, state, and national dental programs.
2. Public health programs offer public education and prevention-oriented programs.

B. Endodontics is the specialty concerned with the treatment of pulpal and periapical diseases of the teeth

1. Diagnostic tests include percussion, palpation, mobility, and use of the vitalometer-pulp vitality tester
2. Reamers enlarge and measure the length of the root canal
3. Files decrease root diameter
4. Broaches remove nerve debris from the root canal
5. Canals are irrigated and then dried with paper points
6. **Obturation** or filling of the canal is done with gutta percha
7. Endodontic condensers or spreaders are used to condense the gutta percha and seal the apex

C. Oral pathology treats the abnormal conditions and diseases of the oral cavity and maxillofacial structures.

1. Biopsy, a minor surgical procedure, is done to remove a specimen from the suspicious lesion
2. Developmental disturbances such as cleft lip, or cleft palate may be treated by the oral pathologist
3. Test results are reported in a formal lab report

D. Oral and Maxillofacial Surgery

1. Oral surgery requires treatment of pain and anxiety through anesthesia either local or general
2. **Sedation** may be required during maxillofacial surgical procedures
3. Treatment of oral cancer is the responsibility of the oral surgeon
4. Most common oral surgery procedure is the simple extraction
5. Complicated procedures involve treatment for fractures of the mandible or maxilla
6. Postoperative instructions may include postoperative antibiotic therapy

E. Orthodontics is the study of the growth and development of the jaw and face

1. **Malocclusions** develop as a result of factors such as face form, jaw relation, and the position and size of teeth

---

ORTHODONTIC CHAIRSIDE DENTAL ASSISTANT MUST BE ABLE TO SELECT AND PREPARE DENTAL INSTRUMENTS FOR THE FOLLOWING ORTHODONTIC PROCEDURES

Adapting extraoral headgear	Impressions	Placement/removal brackets
Appliance construction	Occlusal registrations	Placement/removal fixed appliances
Archwire formation	Oral prophylaxis	
Bonding procedures	Orthodontic adjustments	Placement/removal ligatures
Cementing procedures/removal	Orthodontic emergencies	Placement/removal separators
Cephalometric tracing	Photographs	Radiographs
Diagnostic casts	Placement/removal archwires	Repair removal appliances
Fluoride treatment	Placement/removal bands	Splints

2. Diagnostic tools for classifying occlusion include clinical examination, health history, tooth relationships, plaster study models, bite records, cephalometric radiographs
3. Edward H. Angle's classification of occlusion
   a. normal or neutral occlusion—ideal
   b. **Class I malocclusion** has normal molar relationships with other alterations such as crossbites, rotated teeth, overbites
   c. **Class II malocclusion** has a distal relationship of the mesiobuccal groove of the mandibular first permanent molar to the mesiobuccal cusp of the maxillary first permanent molar
      1) **Class II—Division I** has protruded maxillary anterior teeth
      2) **Class II—Division II** has one or more maxillary teeth retruded
   d. **Class III malocclusion** has a mesial relationship of the mesiobuccal groove of the mandibular first permanent molar to the mesiobuccal cusp of the maxillary first permanent molar
4. When molars are missing the canines are used to determine inter-arch relationships (refer to Chapter 2, Dental Anatomy—Occlusion)

F. Pedodontics the area of dentistry concerned with the prevention, diagnosis and treatment of children's dental problems
1. Thumbsucking is a common oral habit of children
2. Eruption patterns and health of permanent dentition should be closely monitored

G. Periodontics is the specialty concerned with the hard and soft tissues that support the teeth
1. Primary cause of periodontal disease is bacteria in dental plaque
2. Plaque will calcify and form into calculus if not removed
3. Gingivectomy refers to removal of gingival tissue, and gingivoplasty indicates reshaping
4. Surgical **dental implants** may be performed by the periodontist to replace missing teeth
5. Endosteal implants are embedded into the bone
6. Titanium is a treated metal used to form an implant screw or cylinder
7. **Osseointegration** integrates the implant directly into the underlying bone
8. Plastic instruments designed for cleaning implants is preferred

H. Prosthodontics involves the replacement of missing teeth in partially or fully edentulous mouths
1. **Fixed prosthetic appliances** cannot be removed once cemented
2. Final impressions are sent to the dental laboratory where cast frameworks are fabricated
3. Full dentures are required if the mouth is completely edentulous
4. Partial dentures may be fabricated if the remaining teeth can support the forces of mastication

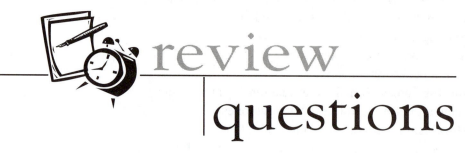

review questions

DIRECTIONS Each of the questions or incomplete statements below is followed by suggested answers or completions. Select the **one answer** that is best in each case.

1. A cavity preparation that includes the mesial incisal angle of a maxillary central incisor is classified as a
   A. Class I cavity preparation.
   B. Class II cavity preparation.
   C. Class III cavity preparation.
   D. Class IV cavity preparation.

2. In application of the rubber dam, which tooth should be used as the anchor tooth?
   A. the tooth being prepared
   B. the opposing tooth being prepared
   C. one or two teeth distal to the tooth being prepared
   D. one or two teeth mesial to the tooth being prepared

3. Protective barriers are necessary when
   A. filing dental records.
   B. sterilizing instruments.
   C. reviewing a dental treatment plan.
   D. mounting x-rays.

4. During the administration of local anesthesia aspiration will
   A. damage the mandibular inferior alveolar nerve.
   B. numb the trigeminal nerve branch.
   C. determine if the lumen of the needle is in a blood vessel.
   D. cause the needle to bend.

5. The reading that is recorded first when taking blood pressure is the
   A. systolic measurement.
   B. diastolic measurement.
   C. pulse measurement.
   D. respirations per minute.

6. The assistant holds the hand instrument to be transferred between the
   A. thumb and forefinger.
   B. small finger and palm.
   C. ring finger and small finger.
   D. thumb and ring finger.

7. The matrix band should be removed
   A. firmly with a serrated hemostat.
   B. quickly with a teasing motion.
   C. slowly in an occlusal or incisal direction.
   D. quickly through the sulcus.

8. Which of the following is NOT a hand cutting instrument?
   A. gingival margin trimmer
   B. hoe
   C. chisel
   D. beavertail burnisher

9. When taking an alginate impression of the upper arch the patient should be seated in a (an)
   A. slightly reclined position with the chin tilted downward.
   B. upright position with head tilted forward.
   C. upright position with head tilted back.
   D. supine position.

10. To ensure that the set alginate impression remains firmly attached in the tray during removal from the mouth the assistant should select a
    A. water-cooled tray.
    B. perforated or rim-lock tray.
    C. compound custom made tray.
    D. acrylic resin disposable tray.

11. A temporary filling is best packed with a
    A. plastic spatula.
    B. moist cotton pellet.
    C. condensor.
    D. spoon excavator.

12. Which of the following statements is true concerning placement of a wedge for a matrix?
    A. It must separate the teeth slightly.
    B. It is used only in conjunction with the rubber dam.
    C. It is placed in the smallest embrasure.
    D. It must extend at least 3 millimeters below the gingival margin.

13. Before application of a topical anesthetic the area should be
    A. examined with a explorer.
    B. dried with a 2× 2 gauze square.
    C. wiped with an alcohol gauze square.
    D. dried for an x-ray exposure.

14. What instruments are best suited for removing excess cement from the teeth?
    A. low-speed handpiece with polishing cup
    B. dental floss and periodontal probe
    C. condensers and carvers
    D. explorer and scaler

15. Endodontic files are used
    A. to enlarge the root canal.
    B. to remove the contents of the pulp chamber.
    C. as drains in an endodontic abscess.
    D. to reduce the occlusal forces of an endo-donticallly treated tooth.

16. A postextraction dressing can be used
    A. on a periodontal surgical site.
    B. only in impacted third molar extraction sites.

    C. if exudate is present.
    D. when there is loss of the blood clot in an extraction site.

17. On the nitrous oxide unit, the flowmeter
    A. indicates the pressure of gas within the cylinder.
    B. controls the breathing bag gas reservoir flow.
    C. provides operator with a guide to the flow of volume of gas to patient.
    D. transports gas from unit to mask.

18. When applying pit and fissure sealants, it is best to
    1. use zinc phosphate cement for etching.
    2. use protective eyewear if light cured.
    3. test occlusion and interproximal contacts.
    4. apply a rubber dam or isolate with cotton rolls.
    A. 1, 4
    B. 2, 3
    C. 2, 4
    D. 1, 2, 3
    E. 2 only

19. When cementing temporary crowns
    1. it is best to use a temporary cement.
    2. a thick insulating base is placed in the crown prior to seating.
    3. the occlusion is checked after cementation.
    4. it is best not to use dental floss to clear the contacts.
    A. 1, 2
    B. 1, 3
    C. 2, 4
    D. 1, 2, 3
    E. All of the above

20. The mouth mirror may be used to
    1. retract the cheeks.
    2. retract the tongue.
    3. reflect light.
    4. provide indirect vision.
    A. 1, 2
    B. 1, 3
    C. 2 only
    D. 3 only
    E. all of the above

✓ answers & rationales

1.
D. Class IV cavity preparations involve the proximal surface and the incisal angle of incisors and canines.

2.
C. When applying a rubber dam, the anchor tooth (tooth that is clamped) selected is one or two teeth distal to the tooth being prepared.

3.
B. Protective barriers are necessary when sterilizing instruments. Heavy-duty utility gloves should be worn when handling soiled armanentarium and scrubbing instruments before sterilization. A face mask and safety glasses also may be used.

4.
C. The purpose of aspiration is to find out if the lumen of the needle is in a blood vessel. If blood is aspirated, the needle is moved to another location before the local anesthetic is deposited.

5.
A. The reading that is recorded first when taking blood pressure is the systolic measurement. Systolic blood pressure is the pressure exerted on the walls of arteries when the heart contracts. In healthy young adults, the average blood pressure is 120/80. The measurement is recorded as a fraction, with 120 representing the systolic measurement and the number 80 representing the diastolic measurement.

6.
A. When transferring an instrument, the assistant holds it between the thumb and forefinger, parallel to the instrument being used, close to the operating field, and opposite the working end, which is pointed toward the surface at which it will be used.

7.
C. The matrix band is removed slowly and carefully teased off the tooth in an occlusal direction. As the matrix band becomes free, the marginal ridge of the amalgam restoration must be held in place with an instrument to avoid accidental fracture of the restoration during matrix band removal procedures. If working on an anterior tooth the matrix band is removed incisally.

8.
D. The beavertail burnisher is not a handcutting instrument. The primary function of a burnishing instrument is to smooth out a metal surface while it is still malleable. The spoon excavator is used to remove soft carious dentin from a cavity preparation, and the hoe and gingival margin trimmer are used to bevel and redefine a cavity preparation.

9.
B. To prevent gagging or excess flow of alginate impression material down the back of the throat, the patient should be seated in an upright position with the head tilted slightly forward.

10.
B. The appropriate trays for obtaining alginate impressions are perforated Rim-lock (autoclavable) trays or perforated plastic (disposable) trays. Water-cooled trays are used for final hydrocolloid impressions, and styrofoam disposable trays are

used for fluoride treatments. Custom-made dental compound trays are best suited for edentulous impressions with a zinc-oxide eugenol impression paste material.

11.

C. A temporary filling is best packed (filled) with a condenser type of instrument. The appropriate condenser should be selected to adapt to the size of the cavity preparation.

12.

A. Criteria for a properly placed wedge (either wooden or plastic) requires that the wedge ensure stability of the matrix band and separate the adjacent teeth slightly.

13.

B. A topical anesthetic is used before administration of a local anesthetic injection for temporary surface numbness of the oral tissues. The oral tissue is dried with a 2×2 gauze before applying the topical anesthetic agent.

14.

D. The best instruments for removing excess cement from teeth are a scaler and an explorer. Dental floss is effective for removing residual cement debris from interproximal surfaces. A knot may be formed in the dental floss before running the floss interproximally for removal of embedded deposits.

15.

A. Three endodontic instruments are used in the root canals: *files* are used to enlarge and shape the canal, *broaches* are used to remove pulpal tissue from the canal, and *reamers* are used to check the path and length of the canal.

16.

D. A dry socket (alveolar osteitis) is a breakdown of a blood clot in an extraction socket. It may be caused by infection, poor blood supply to the area, excessive trauma during extraction or improper postoperative care. Treatment of a dry socket consists of irrigation of the socket and packing it with gauze and an anodyne.

17.

C. The flowmeter controls the volume of gas administered to the patient. The flow of each gas—oxygen and nitrous oxide—is indicated in liters per minute when regulated by the control dials. By observing the positions of the floats in the flowmeter columns of each cylinder gauge, it is possible for the operator to determine the appropriate volume of gas necessary for effective sedation and dental treatment.

18.

C. During the application of pit and fissure sealants, which are polymerized by an ultraviolet light, it is necessary to use protective shaded eyewear. In order to keep the teeth as dry as possible before sealant application, a rubber dam may be applied.

19.

B. When cementing temporary crowns, the consistency and amount of cement placed in the temporary crown depends on the type of crown to be seated. After cementation, the occlusion is checked and adjusted.

20.

E. The mouth mirror may be used to retract the buccal mucosa and tongue and to reflect or illuminate light in the oral cavity. The mouth mirror is used for indirect vision while working on the lingual surfaces of the maxillary anterior teeth and in other areas where direct vision is not possible.

Dental Radiology

➤ Basic Principles of Radiology

➤ Radiation Effects and Safety

➤ Radiographic Exposures

➤ Film Packets

➤ Types of Intraoral Radiographs

➤ Extraoral Films

➤ Panoramic Radiography

➤ Techniques of Intraoral Radiography

➤ Standard Full-Series Radiograph Surveys

➤ Rules for Exposing Radiographs

➤ Development Process

➤ Steps for Mounting Radiographs—Landmarks

➤ Infection Control and Radiographs

contents

Through the diligent work of leaders in the scientific field and through advanced technology, x-ray films have become an important and sophisticated diagnostic tool in dentistry. This chapter presents an overview of the principles of x-ray production, x-ray film processing techniques, methods of evaluation in identifying exposure errors, and occupational radiation safety.

KEY TERMS

ALARA	Fixer
Bisecting	Inverse Square Law
Bitewing	Kilovolt Peak (KVP)
Collimation	Millampere (MA)
Contrast	Periapical Radiograph
Density	Primary Radiation
Exposure Time	Radiolucent
Film Badge	Radiopaque
Focal Film Distance	Secondary Radiation

Characteristic Properties of X-rays

Have no mass
Are not perceptible to the senses
Travel in straight lines
Are not seen in the visible light spectrum
Are capable of producing images on photographic film
Can ionize atoms or molecules
Are capable of causing biologic changes in the person exposed to radiation
Are used in high concentrated doses on human tissue to destroy tumors in the treatment of cancer

Basic Components for X-ray Production

Cathode and tungsten filament to supply electrons
High voltage to accelerate electrons
Anode or target on which electrons are focused and interact to generate x-rays

I. BASIC PRINCIPLES OF RADIOLOGY

A. X-rays belong to a group of radiations called electromagnetic radiations
   1. X-rays are manufactured and have short wavelengths
   2. Short wavelengths give off high energy
   3. X-rays travel through solid objects and penetrate dense tissues, including bone

B. Characteristic properties of x-rays
   1. X-rays have no mass (weight) and are not perceptible to any of the senses
   2. X-rays travel in straight lines and cannot be seen in the visible light spectrum
   3. X-rays are capable of producing images on photographic film
   4. X-rays can ionize atoms or molecules
   5. X-rays are capable of causing biologic changes in the persons exposed to them
   6. X-rays in high concentrated doses are used on human tissue to destroy areas of neoplastic cells (tumors) in the treatment of cancer

C. There are three basic components necessary for the production of x-rays in an x-ray tube (Figure 6–1)
   1. Cathode and tungsten filament to supply the electrons
   2. High voltage to accelerate or speed up the electrons
   3. Anode or target (focal spot), on which the electrons are focused and where they interact to generate x-rays
   4. X-rays are produced when electrons strike the target

D. Primary radiation refers to the main beam of x-ray energy emitted from the x-ray tubehead; primary radiation records an image on the x-ray film

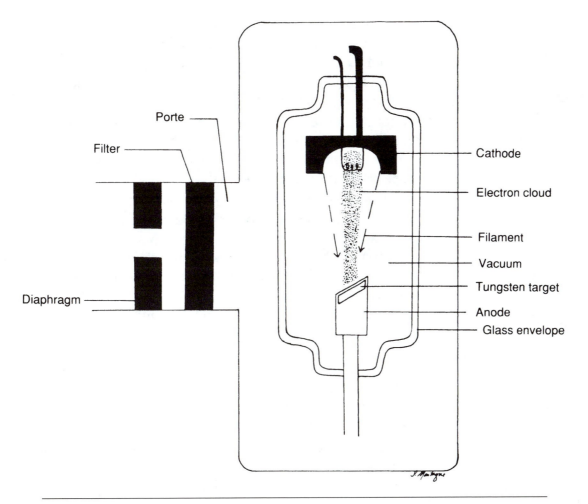

FIGURE 6–1. Diagram of x-ray tube head.

E. Secondary radiation occurs when primary radiation collides with matter
1. Scattered radiation is a form of secondary radiation
2. Scattered radiation denotes x-ray beams that have traveled or have been deflected in all different directions
3. Scatter radiation is difficult to confine and may be scattered throughout the dental operatory

F. Collimation limits the size of the x-ray beam
1. Collimation is accomplished by the use of a lead diaphragm
2. Limits the size of the x-ray beam located within the x-ray tube

G. X-ray unit parameters controlled by the operator
1. Quality (penetrating power) of the x-ray beam, expressed as **kilovolt peak (kVp)**
2. Quantity (number) of x-rays produced, expressed as **millamperage (mA)**
3. Length of time the x-rays are produced, expressed as **exposure time**
4. Suitable penetrating power for dental x-rays ranges from 50 kVp to 100 kVp and 5 mA to 15 mA

> ### X-ray Unit Parameters Controlled by the Operator
>
> Quality—kilovolt peak (kVp) penetrating power of the x-ray beam.
> Quantity—milliamperage (mA) number of x-rays produced.
> Exposure time—length of time x-rays are produced.

II. RADIATION EFFECTS AND SAFETY

A. **Cells most sensitive to radiation are young growing cells, reproductive cells, and blood-forming cells**
1. Young growing cells are found in the pregnant dental patient
2. Cell sensitivity to radiation exposure varies with cell types

B. **National Council on Radiation Protection establishes specific radiation limits for operators of radiation equipment**
1. Maximum permissible dose (MPD) for occupational exposure is 5 rem per year or 0.1 rem per week.
2. Radiation safety includes limitation of radiation exposure

C. **Protective measures for radiation safety involve both time and distance factors**
1. Time factor represents the total history of radiation exposure.
   a. Operator must consider patient's past history of radiation exposure
   b. Number of films needed to obtain diagnostic information
   c. kVp
   d. Exposure time
   e. Film speed
2. Distance factors affect the intensity of the x-ray beam
3. **Inverse Square Law** states that the intensity of the primary beam decreases in proportion to the square of the distance from the source

D. **Radiation can produce both short-term and long-term effects**
1. Latent period is used to describe the time lapse from x-ray exposure until there is observable damage
2. Short-term effects (acute) result from very high doses of radiation as from a nuclear accident
3. Long-term effects occur years after exposure
4. Long-term effects of radiation exposure may include:
   a. Reddening of the skin
   b. Hair loss
   c. Split fingernails
   d. Blindness
   e. Sterility

E. **Radiation protection guidelines recommend adoption of the concept of "ALARA"**
1. **ALARA** stands for "as low as reasonably achievable"
2. Reminds the operator that every dose of radiation produces damage and should be kept to the minimum necessary to meet an appropriate diagnosis

F. **Radiation exposure to the patient is minimized by the following procedures:**
1. Follow federal regulations and guidelines when purchasing x-ray units
2. Periodically check x-ray machines for leakage
3. Check machines to ensure that filters and collimators are placed properly
4. Drape patients with lead lap aprons and thyroid cervical collars (Figure 6–2)

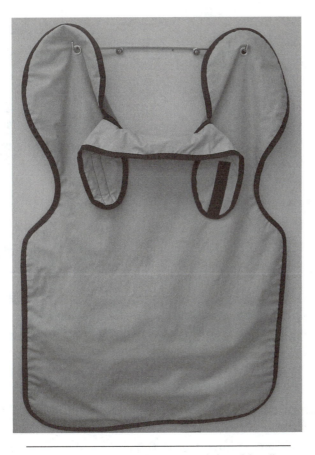

FIGURE 6–2. Lead apron and thyroid collar.

5. Use fast-speed film
6. Employ lead-shielded open-ended cones/tubes, position indicator devices (PID) which reduce scattered radiation
7. Avoid retakes

G. Radiation exposure to the operator is minimized by the following steps
   1. Stand at least 6 feet away, behind a lead shield, or both
   2. Do not hold the film for a patient during an exposure
   3. Use film holding devices for film placement
   4. Personnel should wear **film badges** that periodically monitor dosages
   5. No working area should be in the direct line of the x-ray machine

III. RADIOGRAPHIC EXPOSURES (Figure 6–3)
  A. High-quality radiographs have good density; density is described as the degree of blackness on the radiograph
    1. Number of x-rays that hit the film determines the degree of blackening, or density
      a. **Radiolucent** (black) areas on radiographs are less dense (e.g., pulp chambers, sinus cavities)
      b. **Radiopaque** (white) areas on radiographs are denser (e.g., bone and metallic restorations)

To Minimize Radiation Exposure for the Operator

Stand at least 6 feet away or behind a lead shield
Do not hold the film for a patient during an exposure.
Use film holding devices for film placement
Film badges must be worn for monitoring dosages
Do not place working area in direct line of the x-ray machine

---

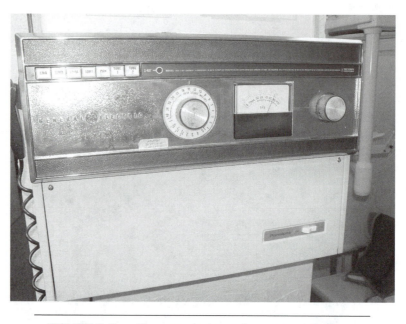

FIGURE 6–3. X-ray control panel: exposure settings.

B. **Range of shades from white to black including all shades of gray is called contrast**
   1. Increasing the kilovoltage (kVp) darkens the radiograph and decreases contrast
   2. Decreasing the contrast lightens the radiograph and produces more shades of gray

C. **Milliamperage and exposure time work together to determine the amount of radiation produced**
   1. Increasing the milliamperage darkens the radiograph and increases the **density**
      a. Contrast is slightly increased and produces fewer shades of gray
      b. Density of radiographs is best controlled by adjusting milliamperage
   2. Changes in exposure time affect density
      a. Increasing the exposure time increases the density and darkens the radiograph
      b. Decreasing the exposure time decreases density and lightens the radiograph

D. **Focal-film distances (FFDs) most commonly used in dentistry are 8, 12, and 16 inches (Figure 6–4)**

IV. FILM PACKET

A. **X-ray film packets consist of a waterproof outer covering, black paper, film, and lead foil**
   1. Lead foil absorbs unused radiation
   2. Foil backing serves to reduce background scatter and prevents film fogging

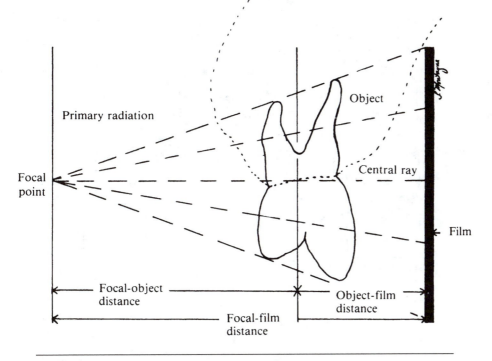

FIGURE 6–4.   Relationship among focal point, object, and film.

B. Film is composed of a silver halide emulsion, covered by gelatin, on a cellulose acetate film
1. Size of silver halide crystals determines the film speed or sensitivity
2. Film speed affects the amount of radiation and the length of time (milliamperes) required to produce an image on the film

C. Film speed will determine how much radiation and exposure time is necessary to produce an image on a film
1. Film speed classification is designated by the American National Standards Institute (ANSI) by letter groups A through F
2. Fast films D through E are used most often in the dental office combining fast-film speed with an acceptable level of detail
3. E film is replacing D-speed film
4. The E-speed film requires one-half the exposure time of D-speed film

D. Film is manufactured in sizes 0 to 4 (Figure 6–5)
1. Periapical film is available in sizes 0, 1, 2
2. Bitewing film is available in sizes 0, 1, 2, 3
3. Occlusal film is available in size 4

E. Store dental films in a lead-lined container so that they are not exposed to scatter radiation, moisture contamination, heat, chemicals, or light
1. Periodic test film runs are recommended to ensure x-ray film quality
2. Outdated films may compromise the diagnostic value of the x-ray

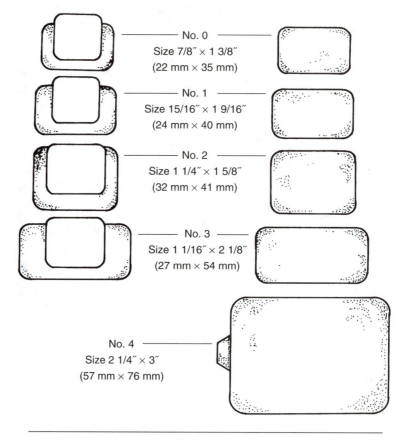

No. 0
Size 7/8″ × 1 3/8″
(22 mm × 35 mm)

No. 1
Size 15/16″ × 1 9/16″
(24 mm × 40 mm)

No. 2
Size 1 1/4″ × 1 5/8″
(32 mm × 41 mm)

No. 3
Size 1 1/16″ × 2 1/8″
(27 mm × 54 mm)

No. 4
Size 2 1/4″ × 3″
(57 mm × 76 mm)

FIGURE 6–5. Film sizes.

V. TYPES OF INTRAORAL RADIOGRAPHS

A. Periapical radiographs show the entire tooth or teeth from the incisal/occlusal edge to the apex (Figure 6–6)

1. Periapical radiographs provide diagnostic information
2. Conditions of the alveolar bone and teeth, presence of infection may be observed

B. Bitewing radiographs show upper and lower teeth in occlusion

1. Provide information useful in detecting the presence of interproximal caries
2. Used to detect periodontal disease (Figure 6–7)
3. Vertical bitewings used to examine alveolar bone level

C. Occlusal radiographs are used to survey larger areas of the jaw (Table 6–1; Figures 6–8 & 6–9)

VI. EXTRAORAL FILMS

A. Extraoral films are radiographs taken with the film outside the patient's mouth (Table 6–2; Figures 6–10 to 6–12)

1. Film size varies
   a. 5 × 7 inches
   b. 8 × 10 inches
   c. 5 × 12 inches

Indicators for Occlusal Radiographs

Locate supernumerary teeth
Locate jaw fractures
Record changes in size and shape of dental arches
Minimize number of x-rays during pedodontic survey
Determine shape and extent of neoplastic cysts
Detect salivary gland calcifications
Locate impacted teeth, retained roots, foreign bodies
Used for patients unable to open mouth wide enough for periapicals

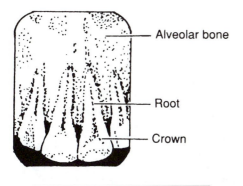

Alveolar bone

Root

Crown

FIGURE 6–6.   Periapical film.

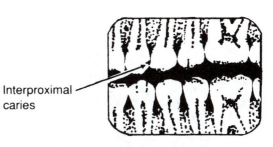

Interproximal
caries

FIGURE 6–7.   Bitewing film.

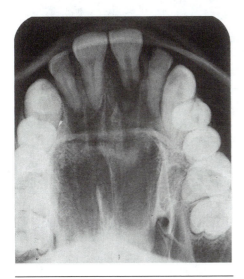

FIGURE 6–8.   Maxillary occlusal radiograph. (Courtesy of Cerritos College Dental Assisting Department.)

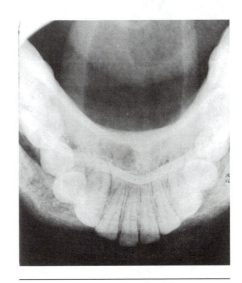

FIGURE 6–9.   Mandibular occlusal
radiograph. (Courtesy of Cerritos College Dental Assisting Department.)

TABLE 6–1   FEATURES OF OCCLUSAL FILMS

ARCH	FILM PACKET PLACEMENT	DIRECTION OF CENTRAL RAY
Maxillary	On occlusal surfaces of maxillary teeth; patient bites down on film packet	Perpendicular to film packet; cone is 2–4 inches away from face; occlusal plane parallel to floor
Mandibular	On occlusal surfaces of mandibular teeth; patient bites down on film packet	Beneath mandible; perpendicular to film packet; cone is 2–4 inches away from face; inferior border of mandible aligned perpendicular to floor

TABLE 6–2   EXTRAORAL FILMS

TYPE OF FILM	AREA VISUALIZED
Lateral skull	Whole skull pathologic survey
Anterior-posterior	Anterior-posterior plane of skull fracture survey
Water's view	Sinuses
Lateral oblique of mandible	One side of mandible, usually for third molar impaction
Temporomandibular (TMJ)	TMJ in various positions
Cephalometric (usually a lateral skull plate)	Identifies anthropometric landmarks essential to orthodontic diagnosis

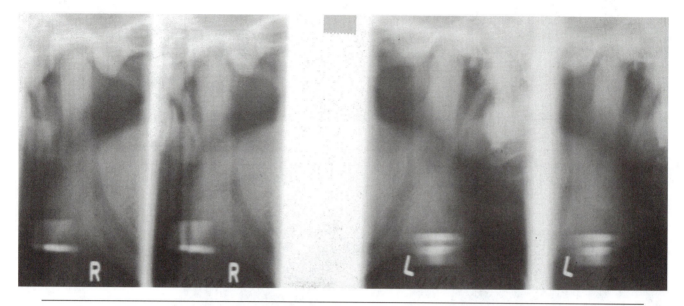

FIGURE 6–10. Extraoral film of temporomandibular joint. (Courtesy of Veterans Administration Medical Center, West Los Angeles.)

2. Films are held in metal/plastic cassettes that perform the same function as the film packet
3. Intensifying screens in the cassettes are used to intensify the radiation and, therefore, decrease the exposure time

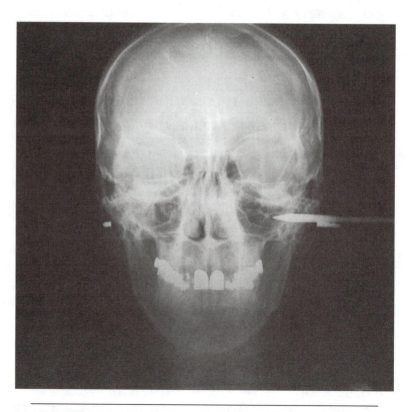

FIGURE 6–11. Cephalometric film (frontal view). (Courtesy of Veterans Administration Medical Center, West Los Angeles.)

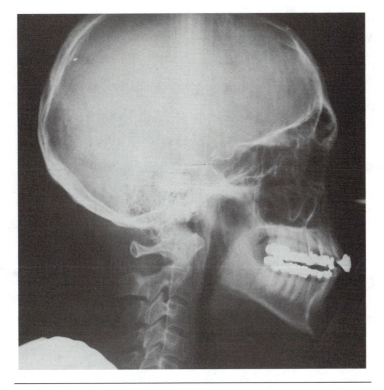

FIGURE 6–12. Cephalometric film (lateral view). (Courtesy of Veterans Administration Medical Center, West Los Angeles.)

VII. PANORAMIC RADIOGRAPHY

A. Panoramic radiography is used to obtain an image of the upper and lower jaw (Figure 6–13)

1. Patient's head is fixed and the x-ray tube and film focus and rotate around the patient's head
2. Film may be used to evaluate facial trauma (fractures) cysts, and tumors
3. Film is useful for assessment of mixed dentition and tooth development and to evaluate the jawbones of the edentulous patient

B. Diagnostic quality includes that the following features be present (Figure 6–14)

1. Condyles, inferior border of the mandible, and maxilla including zygomatic arches, sinuses, and lower portions of both orbits
2. Occlusal plane shows slight upward curve
3. Teeth are same size bilaterally without excessive overlap of interproximal contacts
4. Anterior teeth are of normal size and are not distorted
5. Condyles are approximately equal distance from the top of the film
6. Contrast and density allow visualization of the soft tissue sructures such as the earlobes

C. Advantages of panoramic radiography (Figure 6–15)

1. Areas not seen on a routine full mouth series are shown
2. Both upper and lower teeth are shown on one film
3. Less patient cooperation is required

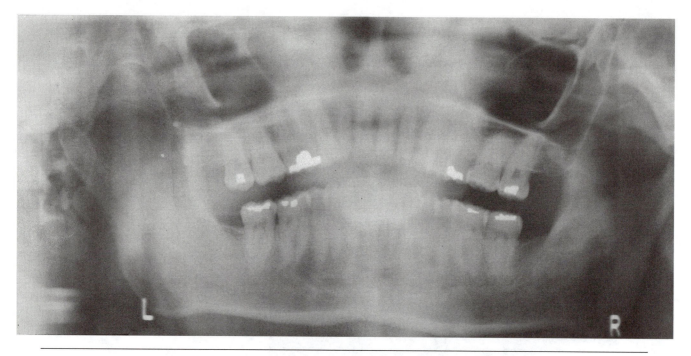

FIGURE 6–13. Panelipse film of adult dentition. (Courtesy of Veterans Administration Medical Center, West Los Angeles.)

4. Gagging is eliminated
5. Less time is required
6. Patient is exposed to a minimum amount of radiation

D. Disadvantages of panoramic radiography
1. Radiograph is not as diagnostic as individual films for caries or bone height
2. Images of teeth are enlarged or distorted

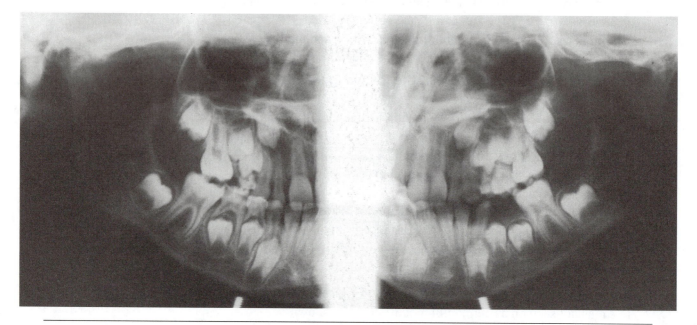

FIGURE 6–14. Panorex film of mixed dentition. (Courtesy of Veterans Administration Medical Center, West Los Angeles.)

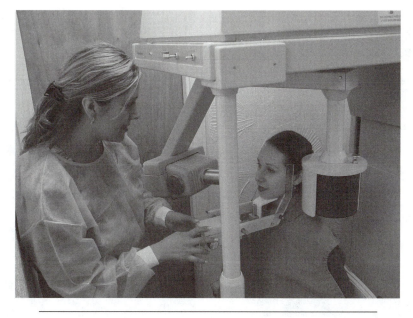

FIGURE 6–15. Pano x-ray machine and operator.

3. Overlapping of contacts in premolars and molars
4. Anterior teeth are difficult to see when they have pronounced inclinations
5. Decreased sharpness and generalized haziness occur

E. Common positioning errors in panoramic radiography include
   1. Improper chin tilt
       a. Chin tilted too far downward (Figure 6–16)
       b. Chin tilted too far upward (Figure 6–17)

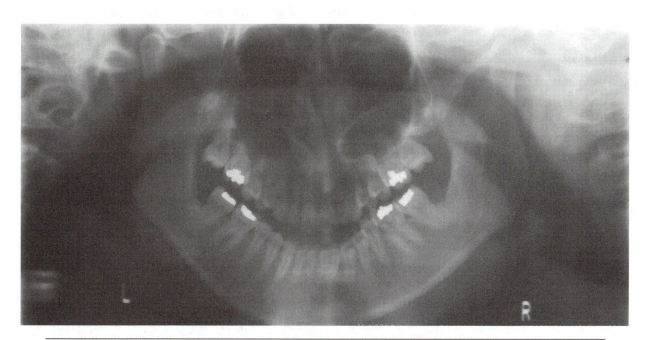

FIGURE 6–16. Chin tilted too far downward. (Courtesy of Veterans Administration Medical Center, West Los Angeles.)

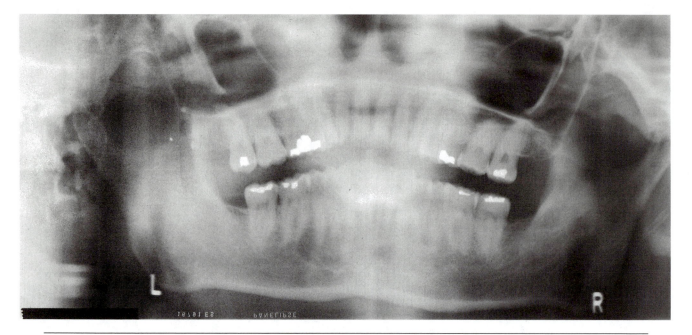

FIGURE 6–17.   Chin tilted too far upward. (Courtesy of Veterans
Administration Medical Center, West Los Angeles.)

2. Noncentered patients
3. Tilting of the head to one side
4. Errors allow structures to appear distorted or projected off the film

VIII.   TECHNIQUES OF INTRAORAL RADIOGRAPHY

A. **Paralleling technique is based on the principle that the object (tooth) and the film are parallel to one another and the central x-ray beam is directed perpendicular to both (Figure 6–18)**
   1. Increased object-film distance results in loss of image detail
   2. Compensate by using a long cone, position indicating device (PID)

B. **Advantages to the paralleling technique**
   1. Image formed on the film will have dimensional accuracy
   2. Owing to minimum distortion, periodontal bone height can be diagnosed accurately
   3. Maxillary molar projection has little or no root superimposition

C. **Disadvantages to the paralleling technique**
   1. Intraoral film-holding devices must be used; may be uncomfortable for the patient
   2. Anatomic features may prevent proper placement of film (e.g., mandibular tori)
   3. Use of a long cone PID necessitates an increase in exposure time

D. **Bisecting the angle technique, an imaginary line is identified that bisects the angle formed by the long axis of the tooth and the film**
   1. Central x-ray beam is directed perpendicular to the imaginary line
   2. Technique uses a short cone position indicating device (Figure 6–19)

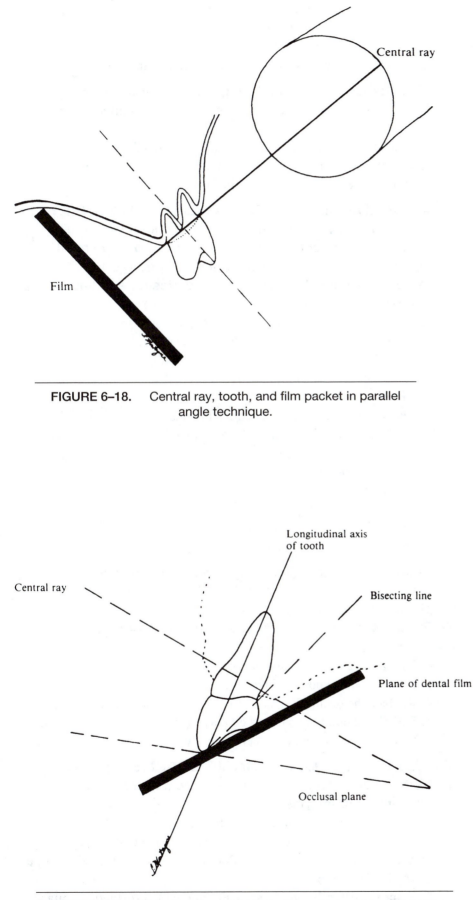

FIGURE 6–18. Central ray, tooth, and film packet in parallel angle technique.

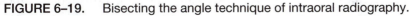

FIGURE 6–19. Bisecting the angle technique of intraoral radiography.

E. Advantages to the bisecting the angle technique
  1. Decreased exposure time
  2. Less cumbersome film holder
  3. Anatomic features usually do not interfere with film placement

F. Disadvantages to the bisecting the angle technique
  1. Image projected on the film is dimensionally distorted in varying degrees
  2. True alveolar bone height can be misinterpreted
  3. Use of a short cone PID results in divergent rays; image is not an optimum reproduction of the object.

IX. STANDARD FULL-SERIES RADIOGRAPH SURVEYS

A. Full-mouth series of radiographs for an adult with a full complement of teeth is usually composed of at least 14 to 16 periapical films and 4 bitewing films (Figure 6–20)
B. Projections constitute a typical full series for a patient with a complete dentition
  1. Maxilllary periapical projections include:
    a. Right and left central and lateral incisors
    b. Right and left canines
    c. Right and left premolars
    d. Right and left molars
  2. Mandibular periapical projections include:
    a. Right and left central and lateral incisors
    b. Right and left canines
    c. Right and left premolars
    d. Right and left molars
  3. Horizontal bitewing projections include:
    a. Right and left premolars
    b. Right and left molars

C. Pedodontic full-mouth survey differs from the adult full-mouth survey in the number of radiographs and the size of film packets used (Figure 6–21)
D. Edentulous full-mouth survey consists of 14 periapical films
  1. Bitewing films are not taken
  2. Increase the vertical angulation
  3. Decrease the exposure time
  4. Replace the occlusal plane with the crest of the edentulous ridge
  5. Pathologic conditions observed may include cysts, abscesses, retained root tips, impacted teeth

X. RULES FOR EXPOSING RADIOGRAPHS

A. Certain rules and procedures must be followed when exposing radiographs
  1. Review patient's medical/dental history
  2. Position patient's head so that the occlusal plane of the jaw being radiographed is parallel to the floor and the midsagittal plane is perpendicular to the floor
  3. Remove patient's eyeglasses and removable prosthetic appliances

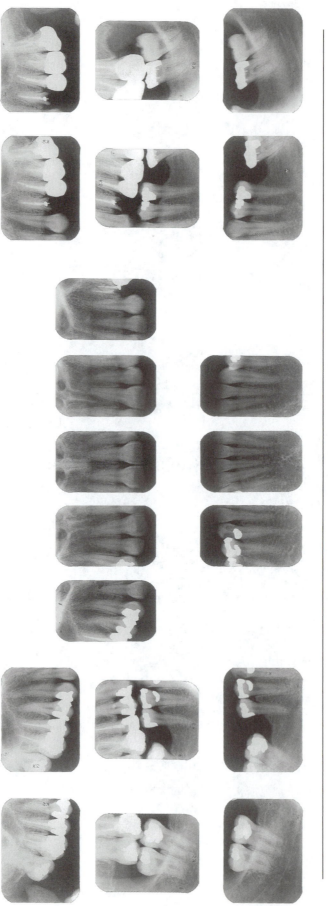

FIGURE 6–20. Adult full mouth survey. (Courtesy of Veterans Administration Medical Center, West Los Angeles.)

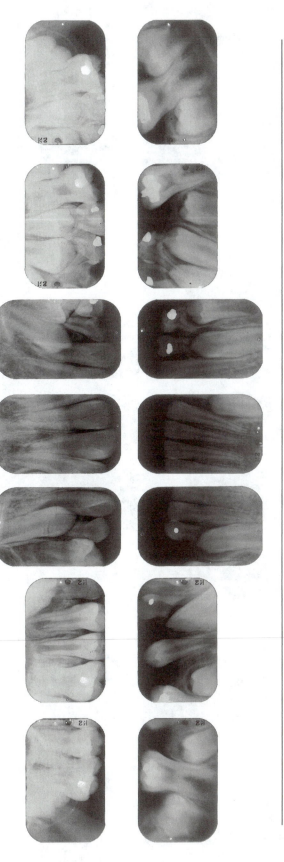

FIGURE 6–21. Pedodontic full mouth survey.
(Courtesy of Cerritos College Dental Assisting Department.)

4. Drape the patient with a lead lap apron that extends from the neck past the genital area and thyrocervical collar
5. Set desired exposure time before placing film in patient's mouth
6. After exposure is made, remove the film from patient's mouth; dry film and place it in a disposable cup
7. Never place films, exposed or unexposed, within an operatory where exposures are made
8. Follow a definite order when taking a full series; do not shift from area to area
9. Use appropriate infection control techniques and protective barriers when exposing radiographs
10. Use PIDs and aiming devices/film holders

B. Common errors in exposure of a full-mouth series of radiographs (Table 6–3)

XI. DEVELOPMENT PROCESS

A. The developing process occurs in the darkroom; darkroom is a separate room used specifically for processing exposed radiographs

B. Following components and requirements are essential for the darkroom
1. No light leaks (films out of their holders are light-sensitive)
2. Safelight
3. Developing tank with three compartments

TABLE 6–3   ERRORS IN EXPOSURE OF FULL MOUTH SERIES OF RADIOGRAPHS

COMMON ERROR	REASONS
Elongation (most common error)	Too little vertical angulation; occlusal plane not parallel to floor; film not against tissue; poor film placement
Foreshortening	Too much vertical angulation; poor chair position
Cone cutting (clear film, curved line)	Beam not aimed at center of film
Film reversal or herringbone effect	Film placed in mouth backward
Film placement	Film not placed far enough in patient's mouth
Saggital plane orientation (occlusal surfaces appear because patient has leaned over; elongation and distortion)	Plane not perpendicular to floor
Overlapping	Incorrect horizontal angulation (central ray not perpendicular to center of film)
Crescent-shaped marks (black lines)	Overbent films; cracked emulsion
Light films (underexposed) (image not dense enough)	Incorrect milliamperes (too low) or time (too short); cone not approximating patient's face; incorrect focal film distance (FFD)
Dark films (overexposed) (image too dense)	Incorrect milliamperes (too low) or time (too long)
Double exposure	Film used twice
Fogged films	Exposure to radiation other than primary beam
Artifacts	Failure to remove prosthetic appliances, earrings, or eyeglasses
Clear films	Unexposed
Blurred image	Caution patient to avoid movement; adjust tube head and extension arm to prevent drifting
Poor contrast	Incorrect, kVp—too high; to correct, decrease kVp

a. Developer—usually on the right
b. Wash
c. Fixer
4. Timing device
5. Thermometer (in developing solution)
6. Rack on which to place films
7. Clean working surface
8. Sink (for cleaning tanks)
9. View box
10. Storage space

C. **Before developing films, all solutions should be stirred to ensure that they are homogeneous and that the temperatures are equalized**
1. Log should be kept noting dates of solution changes
2. Daily recording of solution temperatures is recommended

D. **Appropriate measures must be followed for waste disposal of radiographic processing chemicals**

E. **Film processing is done under safelight conditions in the darkroom**
1. Developing solutions reduce the energized silver halide crystals to silver
2. Films are placed in running water (wash) for 20 to 30 seconds to remove any remaining developing solution
3. **Fixer** removes the unexposed silver halide crystals from the emulsion and preserves the picture
4. Radiographs must be placed in the fixer for a minimum of ten 10 minutes
5. After films are fixed, return to final wash tank for at least 20 minutes
6. Films must be dried in a dust-free, clean area

F. **Common errors made in the darkroom (Table 6–4)**

TABLE 6–4 COMMON ERRORS IN THE DARKROOM	
ERROR	CAUSES
Record keeping	Racks not labeled
Fogged film	White light leak; faulty safelight
Underdeveloped film	Incorrect time (short) and temperature (cold); expended solutions (weak solutions)
Overdeveloped film	Incorrect time (long) and temperature (hot)
Developer cutoff (top of film is clear straight line)	Solutions too low
Clear films (emulsion washed away)	Films left in wash (running rinse water) for more than 24 hours
Stained film	Sloppy or dirty working surface
Scratched film	Racks hit; fingernails too long
Brown films	Films have not had adequate fixation
Torn emulsion	Films touching or overlapping while drying
Static marks (multiple black linear streaks)	Static electricity caused by friction when opening film packet
Lost films	Films not placed carefully in rack

G. Automatic processing equipment saves time and maintains the appropriate time-temperature relationship

1. Machines require periodic cleaning to run smoothly
2. Solutions must be changed regularly

H. Duplicating film has emulsion on one side only; films which have been exposed and previously processed may be duplicated

XII. STEPS FOR MOUNTING RADIOGRAPHS

A. To mount radiographs correctly, refer to anatomic landmarks (Tables 6–5 & 6–6)

1. Separate the films into three piles
   a. Anterior periapicals
   b. Posterior periapicals
   c. Bitewings
2. View the anterior films with the dot facing outward
3. Separate the maxillary films from the mandibular films
4. Mount the anterior periapical films
5. Incisal edges of the maxillary anteriors are to be facing downward
6. Incisal edges of the mandibular anteriors are to be facing upward
7. View the posterior films with the dot facing outward
8. Separate the mandibular films from the maxillary films
9. Mount the posterior periapicals
10. Occlusal surfaces of the maxillary teeth are to be facing downward
11. Occlusal surfaces of the mandibular teeth are to be facing upward
12. View the bitewing films with the dot facing outward
13. Mount the horizontal bitewings; bitewings should match with the crowns of the periapical films directly above
14. Check the mounted radiographs
    a. All dots are facing same direction
    b. All incisal and occlusal surfaces are facing in the proper direction
    c. Radiographs on right side of mount are matching

TABLE 6–5	RADIOLUCENT ANATOMIC LANDMARKS
AREA	**LANDMARKS**
Mandibular molar	1. Mandibular canal (inferior alveolar canal)
	2. Mandibular foramen
Mandibular premolar	1. Mental foramen
	2. Mandibular canal
Mandibular cuspid	1. Mental foramen (position varies)
Mandibular incisor	1. Lingual foramen
Maxillary premolar	1. Anterior portion of maxillary sinus
Maxillary cuspid	1. Nasal fossae
	2. Maxillary sinus
Maxillary incisor	1. Incisive foramen and portion of incisive canal
	2. Median palatine suture
	3. Nasal fossae
	4. Outline of nasal shadow

TABLE 6–6	RADIOPAQUE ANATOMIC LANDMARKS
Area	**Landmarks**
Mandibular molar	1. Anterior border of ramus
	2. External oblique line
	3. Mylohyoid line—internal oblique
	4. Impacted third molar
Mandibular premolar	1. Inferior border of mandible
	2. Mylohyoid line or ridge
	3. Mandibular tori
Mandibular cuspid	1. Mental process
	2. Inferior border of mandible
Mandibular incisor	1. Genial spine or tubercle
	2. Mental prominence
	3. Inferior border of mandible
	4. Mental symphysis
Maxillary molar	1. Coronoid process
	2. Pterygoid hamulus
	3. Zygomatic arch
	4. Maxillary tuberosity
	5. Outline of maxillary sinus
Maxillary premolar	1. U-shaped zygomatic process
	2. Floor of nasal cavity
	3. Outline of maxillary sinus
Maxillary cuspid	1. Inverted Y-formation of maxillary sinus
Maxillary incisor	1. Median nasal septum
	2. Outline of soft tissue of nose

    d. Radiographs on left side of mount are matching
    e. Difference in size of anterior teeth—mandibular anterior teeth are smaller than maxillary anterior teeth
    f. Differing bone densities in the mandibular and maxillary arches
    g. Upward curve of bone at the end of the mandibular arch
    h. Maxillary first premolars usually have two roots whereas mandibular first premolars have one root

B. Mounted radiographs are read by the dentist for interpretation and diagnosis on an illuminated x-ray viewbox
    1. Mounted films are placed in a protective envelope and filed in the patient's dental chart
    2. All x-rays taken must be filed and stored along with the patient's permanent dental record for legal purposes

XIII. INFECTION CONTROL AND RADIOGRAPHS
  A. Infection control practices must be implemented when exposing and processing radiographs
    1. Tube head and exposure control switch must be protected with barrier covers
    2. Personal protective equipment must be worn during patient contact

3. Individual film packets are available in clear plastic barrier envelopes to facilitate infection control protocols in the darkroom
4. Film holding instruments must always be sterilized if they are not disposable
5. After exposing intraoral radiograph wipe the film with a paper towel or gauze to remove saliva
6. Light spray of disinfectant may be used on packet as long as there is no moisture contamination
7. Place exposed film in a disposable paper cup for processing

B. **In the darkroom, carefully unwrap the film packets, spill the untouched film on an uncontaminated flat surface and dispose of the wrappings, including gloves in a waste receptacle**
C. **Surfaces in the darkroom that may become contaminated must be cleaned and disinfected with an approved EPA intermediate-level surface disinfectant agent**
D. **Daylight loaders must not be contaminated with soiled gloves**
   1. Place exposed film in a paper cup and remove soiled glove
   2. Use clean gloved hands to place cup inside the daylight loader and close lid
   3. Pass clean, gloved hands through the light shield to unwrap the film
   4. Drop the film onto the uncontaminated surface inside the loader
   5. Place the soiled film wrapping in the cup
   6. Remove soiled gloves and place them in the paper cup
   7. Place film into the chute for developing

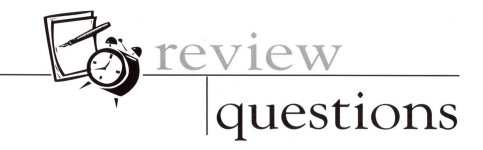

review questions

DIRECTIONS Each of the questions or incomplete statements below is followed by suggested answers or completions. Select the **one answer** that is best in each case.

---

1. X-rays are made up of
   A. electrons.
   B. neutrons.
   C. photons.
   D. anodes.

2. Milliamperage controls
   A. the speed with which electrons move from cathode to anode.
   B. cooling of the anode.
   C. heating of the anode.
   D. heating of the cathode.

3. Collimation of the primary beam
   A. decreases the exposure time.
   B. restricts the shape and size of the beam.
   C. makes the primary beam more difficult to connect.
   D. dictates the contrast of the final radiograph.

4. The lead diaphragm determines the size and shape of
   A. electron cloud.
   B. film used.
   C. x-ray beam.
   D. filament.

5. To increase the penetrating quality of an x-ray beam, the auxiliary must
   A. increase kVp.
   B. decrease kVp.
   C. increase mA.
   D. increase FFD.

6. Filtration of the x-ray beam protects the patient by
   A. eliminating all radiation from the x-ray tubehead.
   B. eliminating weak wavelength x-rays from the x-ray beam.
   C. eliminating short wavelength x-rays from the x-ray beam.
   D. decreasing exposure time.

7. Scatter radiation is a type of
   A. secondary radiation.
   B. primary radiation.
   C. stray radiation.
   D. filtered radiation.

8. The first sign of x-ray dermatitis is
   A. alopecia.
   B. dry skin.
   C. erythema.
   D. itching sensation.

9. The amount of radiation a person receives
   A. begins anew every day.
   B. is cumulative in the entire body.
   C. is not harmful if given in small doses.
   D. comes directly from sunlight and tanning.

10. A technique used to measure the operator's exposure to radiation is
    A. to check the color of the operators hair and fingernails.
    B. to have the operator wear a radiation film badge.

C. to multiply the number of films the operator has exposed by 0.1 rem.

D. to count the number of full mouth x-ray series taken in a week.

11. Accumulated radiation dosage for those who work with radiation may not exceed
    A. 0.1 rem/week.
    B. 1 rem/week.
    C. 10 rems/week.
    D. 100 rems/week.

12. The most effective way to reduce gonadal exposure from x-rays is to
    A. increase the kVp.
    B. use a lead lap apron.
    C. increase vertical and horizontal angulation.
    D. use ultraspeed x-ray film.

13. Film speed is determined by the
    A. amount of silver bromide salts.
    B. thickness of cellulose acetate base.
    C. size of the silver bromide crystal.
    D. color of film packets.

14. The periapical film reveals
    A. the entire jaw.
    B. occlusal surfaces of upper and lower posterior teeth.
    C. lateral views of the skull.
    D. the entire tooth including the apex.

15. The principle used in panoramic radiography is
    A. long cone paralleling principle.
    B. laminagraphy.
    C. tomography.
    D. short cone PIDs.

16. The raised button on the radiograph aids in
    A. determining the film speed.
    B. processing the film in a wet tank.
    C. identifying landmarks that are radiopaque.
    D. mounting radiographs.

17. What is the small circular radiolucency near the roots of the mandibular premolars?
    A. lingual foramen
    B. mental foramen
    C. mandibular foramen
    D. incisive foramen

18. Cone cutting results from the central ray
    A. not being aimed at the center of the film.
    B. having incorrect horizontal angulation.
    C. having increase vertical angulation.
    D. not being aimed at the intensifying screen.

19. Films not fixed for a long enough period of time will appear to
    A. have fine black lines.
    B. be clear.
    C. have a brown tint.
    D. have a thick herring bone pattern.

20. Quality assurance is necessary to ensure that
    1. x-ray film is not outdated.
    2. x-ray units are operating properly.
    3. temperatures are accurate for processing.
    4. test film runs are conducted periodically.
    A. 1 only
    B. 1, 3
    C. 2, 4
    D. 4 only
    E. All of the above

answers & rationales

1.

C. X-rays are made up of bundles of energy called photons. Photons of x-ray frequency are capable of penetrating objects.

2.

D. The milliamperage controls the heating of the cathode and thereby the density of the resultant electron cloud. Increasing the milliamperage will result in a denser cloud and increase in the number of x-rays produced.

3.

B. Collimation of the primary beam restricts its size and shape so it coincides as closely as possible with the size and shape of the film. As the collimated beam approaches the size of the film, there is an increased possibility of cone cutting.

4.

C. The lead diaphragm determines the size and shape of the x-ray beam as it leaves the x-ray head. The distance between the target and the film will determine the size of the beam at the film.

5.

A. The kVp determines the penetrating power of the x-ray beam. Increasing the kVp increases the electrical potential between the cathode and anode. This increases the force driving the electrons from the cathode to the anode, which results in an increase in the penetrating power of the resulting x-ray beam. Dental radiology uses 45 kVp to 95 kVp.

6.

B. Filtration is the passing of the x-ray beam through an aluminum disc to eliminate the longer, weaker wavelength x-rays. Longer wavelength x-rays, also known as soft x-rays, do not have penetrating power and could be absorbed by the patient's cheek.

7.

A. Scatter radiation is a type of secondary radiation created when the primary beam passes through an object.

8.

C. The initial sign of x-ray dermatitis is erythema (redness of the skin).

9.

B. The amount of radiation a person receives is cumulative in the entire body. Therefore, people working with x-rays should take proper precautions to decrease their exposure.

10.

B. An easy way to tell the amount of radiation one is receiving is to wear a radiation film badge. The badge is worn for a period of time, after which the radiation exposure can be measured. If the occupational dose is too high, measures must be taken to correct the problem.

11.

A. The maximum whole-body dose considered permissible is 0.1 rem/week (100 mR/week). Ideally, the operator should receive zero occupational radiation.

12.

B. To prevent gonadal exposure to x-rays, the patient should wear a lead apron. X-rays will not pass through lead. Therefore, the gonadal tissue, which is very sensitive to radiation, will be protected.

13.

C. Film speed is determined by the size of the silver bromide crystals. Larger crystals produce faster film. Faster film requires less total radiation for exposure. Film speed ranges from A to F. Speed range D and E are the fastest and used intraorally. The E-speed film (Ektaspeed) is recommended because it requires one-half the exposure time of D-speed film.

14.

D. Periapical films are used to show the entire tooth and the supporting structures. They come in three sizes: small for children, regular for adults, and narrow for anterior teeth.

15.

B. The principle used in panoramic radiography is laminagraphy. Laminagraphy is the focusing of the x-ray beam at a point that will appear on the resulting film. Other objects in the beam's path are out of focus and do not appear on the radiograph.

16.

D. The button or dot is used to orient the films when mounting. All films should be oriented with the button in the same direction when mounting.

17.

B. The small circular radiolucency near the roots of the mandibular premolars is called the mental foramen.

18.

A. Cone cutting is caused by the central ray not being aimed at the center of the film. This results in part of the film not being exposed to radiation.

19.

C. Film not fixed for a long enough period of time (about 10 minutes) will have a brown tint. Radiographs may be read after a short period of fixing (wet reading) but must be returned to the fixing solution to ensure complete removal of the unaffected silver bromide crystals.

20.

E. Methods of ensuring high-quality x-ray film exposures with minimum radiation exposure for patient and operator include instruments of quality assurance, such as regular monitoring and testing of equipment to prevent malfunctions, regular maintenance of processing solutions, including regulation of solution temperatures, and regular test film runs.

CHAPTER

7

Dental Materials

contents

➤ Properties of Matter

➤ Gypsum Products: Plaster and Stone

➤ Restorative Materials

➤ Composite Resin Materials

➤ Pit and Fissure Sealants

➤ Bonding Agents

➤ Acrylic Resins

➤ Dental Cements

➤ Varnishes and Liners

➤ Dental Porcelain

➤ Bleaching Agents

➤ Impression Materials

➤ Acrylic Denture Base Resins

➤ Custom Trays

➤ Cast Gold Restorations

➤ Abrasive Materials

➤ Endodontic Sedative and Palliative Materials

The science of dental materials includes a wide range of natural and synthetic substances and products used in the delivery of oral health care. This chapter provides a synopsis of dental restorative materials, dental cements, gypsum products, impression materials, endodontic, and sedative dental materials.

KEY TERMS

Acid etch

Alginate

Composite resins

Elastomers

Endothermic

Exothermic

Gypsum

Imbibition

Light cure

Mercury toxicity

Monomer

Polymer

Polymerization

Syneresis

Trituration

I. PROPERTIES OF MATTER
  A. All dental materials are made up of atomic matter that directly affects the chemical and physical working properties of the material
    1. Three different states of matter: solid, liquid, and gas
    2. **Exothermic** reactions give off heat
    3. **Endothermic** reactions absorb heat
  B. Heat is measured in either Fahrenheit or Celsius degrees

II. GYPSUM PRODUCTS: PLASTER AND STONE
  A. The main constituent of all plasters and stones is calcium sulfate hemihydrate
    1. Use of a mask and protective eyewear is recommended to prevent inhalation of fine **gypsum** powders during manipulation
    2. Class I stone is used mainly for pouring casts
    3. Class II stone (high-strength stone) is used to make dies
  B. Water-to-powder ratios (w/p) are important and affect gypsum product setting times (Table 7–1)
    1. The more water added the longer the setting time and the weaker the result
    2. Setting time can be accelerated or retarded by using chemical additives
    3. Length and speed of mixing can affect setting time; a longer more rapid mix will shorten the setting time.

TABLE 7–1   VALUE OF DIAGNOSTIC CAST STUDY MODELS

1. Assist in diagnosis and treatment planning
2. Patient education
3. Record treatment and growth
4. Record tooth form, position, occlusion, and anatomy of restorations
5. Serve as "Before" and "After" diagnostic models

C. **Plasters and stone are mixed in a flexible rubber bowl with a stiff spatula**
   1. A premeasured amount of water is added to the gypsum product
   2. To remove entrapped air bubbles from mix, place mixing bowl on automatic vibrator and vibrate mix well
   3. Add small increments of mixed stone or plaster into an impression to avoid trapping any air
   4. Set impression aside to harden once filled with the stone or plaster

D. **Gypsum materials may be trimmed with a laboratory model trimmer (Table 7–2; Figures 7–1 & 7–2)**
   1. Cast study models are trimmed geometrically and may be polished for esthetics before the patient case presentation appointment.
   2. Dental auxiliaries must use protective eyewear during the trimming procedures and while handling the dry gypsum powder.
   3. Well-ventilated laboratory areas equipped with exhaust systems to minimize prolonged exposure to the gypsum materials are recommended.

III. RESTORATIVE MATERIALS ARE USED FOR PERMANENT RESTORATIONS
A. **Dental amalgam is a combination of a silver-tin alloy with mercury and small amounts of copper and zinc**
   1. The process of mixing together silver alloy particles with liquid mercury is called **trituration**
   2. Trituration may occur by using a mechanical amalgamator
   3. Undertrituration diminishes the properties of amalgam and reduces strength of material
   4. Overtrituration causes the amalgam to be runny in consistency and difficult to manipulate

TABLE 7–2   STEPS FOR TRIMMING AND FINISHING DIAGNOSTIC STUDY CASTS

1. Soak models in water for 5 minutes.
2. Remove any excess material that will interfere with proper occlusion then place wax-bite registration and articulate casts.
3. Apply safety glasses and turn on power and water on model trimmer unit.
4. Trim base of mandibular cast parallel to occlusal plane.
5. Art portion is ⅓ of total height and anatomical portion is ⅔ of total height.
6. Trim heel of mandibular cast, then sides of mandibular cast.
7. Trim front of mandibular cast by rounding anterior cut from cuspid to cuspid.
8. Trim heel of maxillary cast, articulate maxillary and mandibular casts together and note corresponding relation between the heels of the maxillary and mandibular casts.
9. Trim sides of maxillary casts at an angle to heel.
10. Trim front of maxillary anteriors to a sharp point. Point should correspond with midline and extend distally to center of maxillary cuspids.
11. Trim with lab knife to depths of fold and to produce an over-all smooth esthetic appearance. Fill in voids with soft plaster.
12. Allow study casts to dry thoroughly, polish by rubbing with a soft chamois and label with patients name, age, and date.

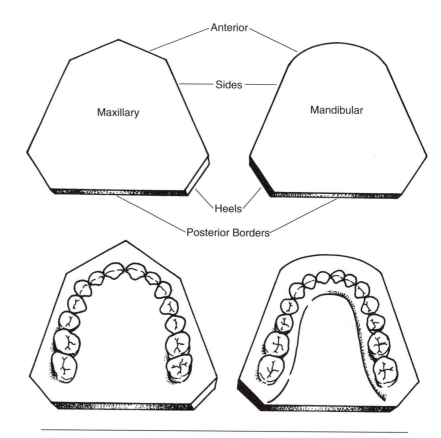

FIGURE 7–1. Trimmed study casts—maxillary and mandibular.

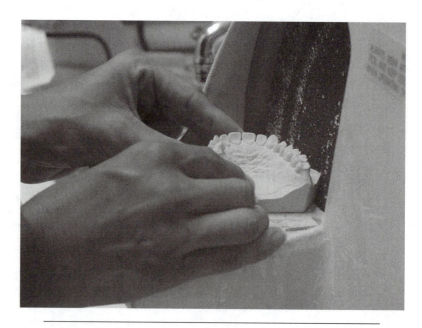

FIGURE 7–2. Trimming and finishing diagnostic study cast.

B. Mercury contamination may occur from accidental spills and direct contact with the liquid metal
  1. Special precautions must be taken by the dental auxiliary when handling mercury to avoid potential occupational and health risks as **mercury toxicity**
  2. Avoid handling fresh alloy and direct contact with mercury
  3. Properly dispose of scrap mercury, preferably in a closed container with a liquid solution
  4. Work in a well-ventilated area of the office when handling mercury materials; use gloves
  5. Pick up spilled mercury immediately with special office emergency spill kits
  6. Use tightly sealed capsules during amalgamation
  7. When removing old amalgam restorations, use the high-speed evacuator and a water spray; masks and face shields should be worn

IV. COMPOSITE RESIN MATERIALS
  A. **Composite resins** are used primarily for anterior restorations; improved resin materials have been developed for use in posterior teeth
  B. Composites exhibit light-cured or self-curing properties
    1. Catalysts quicken setting time
    2. An etchant is applied with an applicator to the preparation
    3. Placement of the mixed composite resin material is done with a plastic placement instrument
    4. Composite resins should not be manipulated with metal instruments
    5. Celluloid matrix strip is used for Class III restorations

V. PIT-AND-FISSURE SEALANTS
  A. Pit-and-fissure sealants are synthetic resins that play an important role in preventive dental procedures; sealants are used to seal pits and fissures
  B. Pit-and-fissure sealants are subject to occlusal wear and must be examined at regular recall intervals

VI. BONDING AGENTS
  A. Enamel bonding agents are used to repair ortho brackets and fractured anterior teeth for esthetics
  B. Dentin bonding agents are used to seal dentinal tubules of a prepared tooth to prevent postoperative sensitivity to the pulp
  C. Before a bonding agent is placed it is necessary to **acid etch** the tooth surface

VII. ACRYLIC RESINS
  A. Acrylic resins are polymeric restorative materials that come in a powder and liquid form
    1. The liquid is a **monomer**
    2. The powder is a **polymer**
    3. Process of curing is called **polymerization**

  B. Acrylic resins may be used for the fabrication of provisional temporary crowns

---

Symptoms of Mercury Toxicity

Chronic headaches
Fatigue
Kidney dysfunction
Tremors
Speech disorders

Dental Cements

Zinc Phosphate Cement
Glass Ionomer
Zinc Oxide Eugenol
Polycarboxylate

VIII. DENTAL CEMENTS IN DENTISTRY—used as luting (cementing or bonding) agents for permanent restorations, orthodontic bands, crowns, and bridges

A. Zinc phosphate cement

1. Zinc phosphate cement is a powder/liquid system
2. Zinc phosphate cement is mixed on a dry, cool glass slab with a metal spatula
3. A thin mix is desired for luting procedures
4. A thick mix is used as an insulating base
5. The material is mixed over a large area of the glass slab in order to dissipate heat
6. The correct consistency for cementation can be determined by checking the flow of the mix

B. Glass ionomer cements

1. Glass ionomer cements come in a powder/liquid form, paste system, and capsule form
2. Glass ionomer cements if in a powder/liquid form are self-curing
3. Glass ionomer cements may be mixed on a nonabsorbent paper pad or a cool glass slab
4. Capsule form of cement material requires use of an amalgamator to triturate
5. Glass ionomer cements with resin-modified formulations are **light-cured**
6. Glass ionomer cements are cariostatic because of their ability to release fluoride ions
7. Luting consistency of glass ionomer cement is creamy
8. Consistency is stiff and tacky when used as an insulating base

C. Zinc-oxide eugenol

1. Zinc-oxide eugenol (ZOE) is dispensed in a powder/liquid or two-paste system
2. ZOE has a sedative effect on the pulp and is used to ameliorate pain from toothaches
3. ZOE may be mixed for temporary crown cementation
4. ZOE is mixed on either a glass slab or paper pad
5. The consistency of ZOE for temporary luting is creamy
6. ZOE has low compressive strength and may be used as a sedative temporary dressing
7. Type II–reinforced ZOE—Intermediate Restorative Material (IRM) serves as a temporary restoration
8. EBA cements are stronger and are used for luting or permanent castings

D. Polycarboxylate cement is a powder/liquid system used for luting or orthodontic band cementation.

1. To increase working time of cement mix on a cool glass slab
2. Failure to mix the cement rapidly will produce a mix with a dull appearance unsuitable for cementation procedures

E. Dental cements are used as thermal insulators for the pulp under metallic restorations.
1. If mixing to a base consistency material must be putty-like
2. Test by rolling material into a ball or cylinder

IX. VARNISHES AND LINERS
A. Varnishes and liners are used to insulate pulpal tissue
1. Application of a varnish may be done with a fine brush or cotton pellet
2. The surface of the preparation is coated with at least two layers of the varnish
3. A varnish does not need to be mixed

B. Calcium hydroxide is a liner which stimulates the formation of secondary dentin
1. Calcium hydroxide is a liner available in liquid/paste or paste/paste form
2. Calcium hydroxide is mixed on a paper pad with a small ball-shaped metal applicator
3. Equal amounts of the base and catalyst are mixed until homogeneous

X. DENTAL PORCELAIN
A. Dental porcelain is an esthetic material widely used in final restorations, crowns, veneers fused to metal copings, and artificial teeth in dentures
B. Tooth shade guides assist in matching the porcelain restoration to the patient's natural dentition

XI. BLEACHING AGENTS
A. Bleaching agents include a high percentage of hydrogen peroxide and may require the use of a curing light
B. In-office bleaching of a non-vital tooth is done when an endodontically treated tooth becomes discolored
C. Home bleaching involves the use of a custom-fitted tray and diluted hydrogen peroxide

XII. ELASTOMERIC IMPRESSION MATERIALS
A. Elastomeric impression materials are self-curing and are available as a base/catalyst system
B. Elastomeric materials polymerize from a paste into a rubber-like impression material
C. Impression material may be premixed and extruded through a cartridge-like syringe or mixed on a mixing pad with a spatula
D. Polysulfide impression material is also known as rubber base
1. The material is supplied in two tubes of paste
2. Used to take final impressions for crowns, bridges, inlays

E. Silicone impression material will polymerize in 6 to 8 minutes

Elastomers
Polysulfide
Silicone
Polyvinylsiloxane
Polyether

F. Polyvinylsiloxane impression material is available as a two-paste system
1. Vinyl gloves are recommended when working with this impression material
2. Materials are dispensed in a specialized impression gun

G. Polyether impression materials are highly accurate and are supplied in tubes with a base and accelerator

XIII. **ELASTIC IMPRESSION MATERIALS (Figure 7-3)**
A. Reversible or agar hydrocolloid is a thermoelastic material used for final impressions
1. Reversible agar hydrocolloids undergo a physical change from sol to gel
2. Water-cooled trays are required for hydrocolloids
3. Hydrocolloid impression materials should be poured immediately
4. **Imbibition** can cause dimensional distortion

B. Irreversible hydrocolloid—alginate
1. Irreversible hydrocolloid—alginate contains seaweed and is supplied as a powder
2. Perforated or rim-locked trays are used for alginate impressions
3. Alginate is mixed in a rubber mixing bowl with a measured amount of room temperature water
4. A metal spatula is used to whip the material into a a homogenous sol
5. Alginate has a low tear strength and will undergo **syneresis** (loss of water) if not stored properly prior to pouring
6. Disinfection measures must be performed when sending alginate impressions to a commercial dental laboratory; use an approved disinfectant to spray the impression
7. Alginate powder contains silica and presents a potential biohazard when inhaled

---

Elastic Impression Materials

Reversible hydrocolloid
Irreversible hydrocolloid—alginate

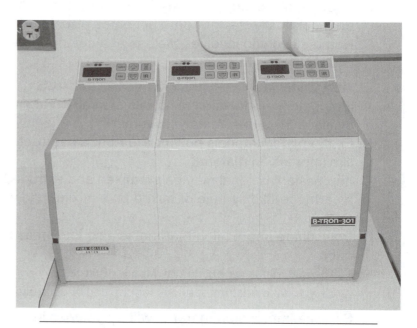

FIGURE 7–3.   Hydrocolloid unit for reversible elastic impression materials.

8. The correct water-to-powder ratios must be used with alginate; setting time affects the strength of the material

9. Algnate is used to take impressions for study models, nightguards, bleaching trays and ortho appliances

XIV. PLASTIC IMPRESSION MATERIALS

A. Dental compound is used to take preliminary impressions for full or partial dentures

1. Dental compound has low thermal conductivity and should be heated slowly and evenly in a waterbath until it can be kneaded

2. Compound sticks are used for single crown preparations

B. Dental waxes

1. Casting wax is used to form the patterns for the metal framework or a removable prosthesis

2. Inlay wax is used to produce patterns for inlays, crowns, and pontics

3. Boxing wax is used to prepare gypsum models

4. Periphery wax is used to adjust impression trays

5. Bite registration is taken using an arch shaped wax

C. Zinc-oxide eugenol (ZOE) impression pastes are used for full denture impressions in a preformed tray

XV. ACRYLIC DENTURE BASE RESINS

A. Self-curing acrylic resins are used to repair dentures that have broken

B. Dentures can be relined if there are minor changes in the oral tissues

C. Cold-cured denture base resins can be used for orthodontic and periodontal splints; occlusal splints for patients with temporomandibular joint dysfunction are also fabricated

XVI. CUSTOM TRAYS

A. Self-cured acrylic resins are used to make custom trays for impressions

1. An electric vacuum former can be used to heat a sheet of plastic material to fabricate custom made bleaching trays, night guards, and protective mouth guards

2. Eliminate all signs of undercuts in the dental cast prior to construction of a custom tray

3. Place appropriate spacer stops to prevent tray from seating incorrectly

4. Fabricate a handle in the anterior part of the tray

5. Separating medium is required during fabrication to facilitate tray removal from the cast

6. Smooth rough tray edges with lab knife and polish

B. Clean tissue side of tray and disinfect before seating in the patient's mouth

XVII. CAST GOLD RESTORATIONS

A. Casting gold alloys are used for inlays, crowns, bridges, and partial denture framework

B. Gold alloy materials are classified according to gold content and hardness which correlates to material strength (Table 7–3)

TABLE 7-3 CLASSIFICATION OF CASTING GOLD ALLOYS
Type I alloys are soft and are used for simple inlays
Type II alloys are harder, can be used for two and three surface inlays, and are the most common alloys used for operative procedures
Type III alloys are used for fixed prostheses, and crown and bridge abutments
Type IV alloys are extra hard and are used for denture frameworks

XVIII. ABRASIVE MATERIALS

A. Caution must be taken if using abrasives in the mouth to prevent overheating the teeth

B. Abrasives and polishing agents can be mixed with a lubricant such as water

C. Dentures are finished by buffing with an abrasive slurry on a laboratory lathe buffing wheel

D. Tin oxide is used for polishing metallic restorations

E. Flour of pumice is used for polishing extrinsic stains from teeth

XIX. ENDODONTIC SEDATIVE and PALLIATIVE MATERIALS

A. Endodontic materials are used to treat the dental pulp and canals of teeth

B. Post-extraction dressings are used as a palliative treatment to alleviate the discomfort of a dry socket (alveolitis)

C. Periodontal dressings are used after periodontal surgery to protect the surgical site from trauma and minimize post-operative discomfort

1. Periodontal dressing materials come as a non-eugenol two-paste system

2. Dressing material is mixed on a paper pad with a tongue depressor

3. Dressing is molded into a thin strip and then gently pressed into the interproximal areas of the surgical site on the facial and lingual surfaces

4. Dressing should not overextend on the occlusal surfaces

5. Provide post-operative instructions to the patient

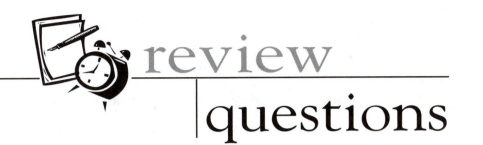

review questions

DIRECTIONS Each of the questions or incomplete statements below is followed by suggested answers or completions. Select the **one answer** that is best in each case.

1. Calcium hydroxide is used primarily as a base to
   A. insulate the pulp thermally.
   B. insulate the pulp chemically.
   C. protect the pulp from bacteria.
   D. promote secondary dentin formation.

2. The chemical used to etch enamel is
   A. eugenol.
   B. zinc oxide.
   C. phosphoric acid.
   D. resin.

3. An impression is a
   A. negative reproduction of oral tissues.
   B. night guard mold.
   C. negative metallic casting.
   D. positive reproduction of a prepared tooth.

4. The impression material capable of change from gel to sol to gel is
   A. silicone.
   B. zinc phosphate.
   C. reversible hydrocolloid.
   D. irreversible hydrocolloid.

5. Which material should be tempered before using?
   A. alginate
   B. reversible hydrocolloid
   C. impression plaster
   D. metallic oxide paste

6. Plaster models
   A. have no dimensional change upon setting.
   B. expand upon setting.
   C. have greater crushing strength than cast stone models.
   D. are thermoplastic.

7. The wax used to make a rim around an impression to contain the poured gypsum material is called
   A. boxing wax.
   B. utility wax.
   C. periphery wax.
   D. blue wax.

8. Acrylic resins are used for
   1. anterior restorations.
   2. temporary bridges.
   3. custom trays.
   4. temporary aluminum crowns.
   A. 1 and 4
   B. 2 and 4
   C. 1, 2, and 3
   D. 2 only
   E. All of the above

9. Advantages of glass ionomer cements include
   1. high adhesion properities.
   2. low abrasion properities.
   3. use as a permanent restoration.
   4. reduction in caries due to fluoride releasing properities.

A. 1, 2
B. 3 only
C. 1, 2, 3
D. 4 only
E. All of the above

10. When trimming study model casts with a model trimmer it is best to
    1. wear protective glasses or face shield.
    2. begin with the mandibular cast.
    3. periodically check casts in occluded position.
    4. allow sufficient water to flow through the model trimmer.
    A. 1, 2, 3
    B. 1, 2, 4
    C. 1, 3, 4
    D. 2, 3, 4
    E. 1, 2, 3, 4

11. Characteristics of pit and fissure sealants may include
    1. self-curing polymerization.
    2. acid etching.
    3. light-cured polymerization.
    4. metallic matrix trips.
    A. 2, 4
    B. 1, 2, 3
    C. 1, 4
    D. 2 only
    E. All of the above

12. The setting time of irreversible hydrocolloid can be altered easily by
    A. using a metallic spatula.
    B. using a perforated tray.
    C. varying the water temperature.
    D. adding distilled water.

13. Imbibition is the
    A. loss of water by hydrocolloid impressions.
    B. increase in model size due to expansion.
    C. decrease in model size due to evaporation of water.
    D. uptake of water by hydrocolloid impressions.

14. Syneresis is the
    A. uptake of water by hydrocolloid impressions.
    B. uptake of water by gypsum products.
    C. loss of water by hydrocolloid impressions.
    D. expansion of elastic impression materials.

15. When using polysulfide impression material, it is necessary to coat the tray with
    A. a separating medium.
    B. petroleum jelly.
    C. a rubber adhesive.
    D. no coating is necessary.

16. Amalgamation is the process of
    A. combining mercury with amalgam alloy.
    B. condensing amalgam into the cavity preparation.
    C. dispensing the amalgam.
    D. burnishing the amalgam against the matrix band.

17. What is the main component of composite restorative materials?
    A. polymethyl methacrylate
    B. hydrogen peroxide
    C. calcium hydroxide
    D. inorganic filler

18. Which of the following statements is TRUE of cavity varnishes?
    A. They may be mixed on a paper pad.
    B. They can be used to seal the dentinal tubules.
    C. They can be used under all restorative materials.
    D. They may be mixed on a glass slab.

19. A periodontal surgical pak is placed
    A. in extraction dry socket sites.
    B. around a dental implant.
    C. directly over sutures at surgical site.
    D. whenever mobile teeth are splinted.

20. Tooth bleaching is a cosmetic procedure for treating teeth with
    A. extrinsic or intrinsic stains.
    B. multiple metallic gold crowns.
    C. porcelain crowns.
    D. erosion or abrasion.

answers & rationales

1.

D. Calcium hydroxide is a base placed beneath deep restorations to promote irritation of the pulp and thereby promote the formation of secondary dentin.

2.

C. Fifty percent solution of phosphoric acid is used to etch enamel. Enamel treated in this manner has increased mechanical retention for resin materials.

3.

A. Impressions are used to fabricate restorations outside the mouth. If a restoration is to fit a tooth (e.g., a crown) and oral tissues (e.g., a denture), the impression must be accurate. An impression is a detailed, accurate negative reproduction of oral tissues. A positive reproduction, or model, which is an exact duplication of the impressed tissues, is obtained by allowing a gypsum product to set in the impression.

4.

C. Reversible hydrocolloid can change from gel to sol and back to gel by heating and cooling. This material can be reused up to four times.

5.

B. To avoid burning the oral tissues, reversible hydrocolloid should be tempered in a water bath at 110°F to 115°F for 5 to 10 minutes before using.

6.

B. All gypsum products expand on setting. Plaster expands more than stone, which expands more than improved stone. Increased expansion may be caused by increased spatulation, increased water/powder ratio, hygroscopic expansion, and the addition of certain chemicals.

7.

A. Stripes of boxing wax are used to form a rim around an impression. This will contain the poured gypsum material and facilitate finishing the model.

8.

C. Some uses of acrylic resins are anterior restorations, bases of full or partial dentures, temporary crowns, and bridges, facings on crowns, prosthetic plastic teeth, bite plates, retainers, custom-made trays, and splints. Advantages of acrylic restorations are that they are insoluble in oral fluids, can be finished in one sitting, are easy to repair and add to the existing restoration, act as a thermal insulator, and are easily manipulated.

9.

E. Glass ionomer cements are very versatile materials that may be used for permanent restorations, luting agents, and thermal base insulators. The glass ionomers exhibit high adhesion properties and low abrasion properties. As a restorative material, the ionomers have the ability to release fluoride ions into the tooth to prevent redecay.

10.

E. When trimming study models with a model trimmer, it is necessary to wear protective eyewear to prevent injury to the eyes. A sufficient water flow must be circulating through the model trimmer unit before use to facilitate the trimming of the plaster/stone models. When actual trimming begins, do not allow fingers to come in close contact with the trimming lathe. Begin by occluding models together and trim the mandibular cast first. After trimming procedures, allow the cast to dry for 24 hours before final polishing and labeling.

11.

B. Characteristics of pit and fissure sealants include self-cured or light-cured polymerization and acid etching. A 35 to 50% solution of phosphoric acid is used to etch the enamel surface. The etching solution cleanses the enamel surface and increases the adherence of the sealant material by creating microscopic openings (pores) on the enamel surface. The resin material then penetrates into the pores and creates a resin bond or tag interlocking the sealant material to the tooth and increasing mechanical retention. Metallic matrix strips are contraindicated.

12.

C. The most effective way to adjust to the setting time of hydrocolloid is to vary the water temperature. Warmer water will accelerate the set; cooler water will retard the set. Changing the at water/powder ratio also will affect the setting time, but it is a poor method because it will weaken the material physically and can alter some of its properties.

13.

D. Imbibition, the uptake of water by hydrocolloid impressions, causes an expansion of the impression. The resulting model will be inaccurate.

14.

C. Syneresis is the exuding of water from hydrocolloid impressions. This loss of water causes shrinkage of the impression, which results in an inaccurate model.

15.

C. When rubber impression materials are used, the tray is coated with a rubber adhesive. Failure to coat the tray can result in the impression separating from the tray.

16.

A. Amalgamation is the combining, chemically and physically, of mercury with amalgam alloy.

17.

D. The main component of composite (sometimes known as filled acrylic resin) is the inorganic filler. The inorganic filler consists of glass particles, fused silica, and quartz crystals. The organic portion of composites is composed of polymers.

18.

B. Cavity varnish is a material that is used to seal the dentinal tubules.

19.

C. Periodontal surgical paks are placed over surgical sites. The periodontal pak or dressing may be placed directly over sutures and is used to protect the tissues during the healing process.

20.

A. Tooth bleaching is implemented primarily for esthetics. The shade of one's teeth may be affected by either extrinsic or intrinsic stains.

8 Infection Control

contents

➤ Modes of Disease Transmission

➤ Universal Precautions

➤ Medical History Data

➤ Hepatitis B Vaccination

➤ Personal Protective Equipment and Barrier Techniques

➤ Handwashing

➤ Sterilization and Monitoring

➤ Disinfection

➤ Dental Laboratory Disinfection

➤ Pre-Treatment Infection Control

➤ Post-Treatment Infection Control

➤ Preparing Instruments for Sterilization

➤ Radiation Asepsis

➤ Management of Office Waste

This chapter will present an overview of basic principle infection-control recommendations and guidelines. Minimizing microbial disease transmission is a key objective in protecting the dental patient and dental health care worker.

KEY TERMS

Aerosol	Pathogens
Asepsis	Personal protective equipment
Biological monitoring	Sepsis
Cross-contamination	Sporicidal
Decontamination	Sterilization
High-level disinfection	Tuberculocidal
Immunization	Universal precautions
Intermediate-level disinfectant	

I. MODES OF DISEASE TRANSMISSION
  A. Infectious microorganisms may be transferred by various methods
   1. Direct contact
   2. Indirect contact
   3. Inhalation—**aerosol** droplets
   4. Contaminated food or water
   5. Cuts or breaks in the skin

  B. **Cross-contamination** can occur if appropriate methods of sterilization, disinfection, and waste disposal are not practiced
II. UNIVERSAL (STANDARD) PRECAUTIONS
  A. **Universal (Standard) Precautions** implies that the same infection control procedures must be used for every patient
  B. Blood and saliva from all dental patients are considered potentially infectious materials
III. MEDICAL HISTORY DATA
  A. Review patient medical and dental health history information prior to the beginning of each treatment session
   1. Health status of each is determined by the health history
   2. Include current questions relative to HIV and HBV

  B. Collect and record data relative to medications and laboratory reports including antibody-antigen test results for infectious diseases.
IV. HEPATITIS B VACCINATION
  A. **Immunization** is the best protection against the hepatitis B virus
  B. Hepatitis B virus is found primarily in blood
   1. Hepatitis B (HBV) can be transmitted through accidental needle sticks
   2. HBV can be found in other body fluids such as saliva, tears, semen, and vaginal fluids

V. PERSONAL PROTECTIVE EQUIPMENT AND BARRIER TECHNIQUES

A. **Personal protective equipment (PPE) is to be worn by employees to reduce the risk of infectious disease transmission**
1. Disposable face mask
2. Protective eyewear or face shield
3. Disposable gloves
4. Clinic jacket/lab coats

B. **Personal protective equipment must not allow blood or other potentially infectious materials to pass through to clothing, skin, or mucous membranes**
1. Change disposable face mask for each patient
2. Replace disposable face mask if mask becomes wet or soiled
3. Protective eyewear should be worn at all times during clinical procedures
4. Protective eyewear protects the eye from flying debris and contamination
5. Protective face shield should be used during clinical procedures that produce aerosol sprays
6. Disposable gloves reduce the potential for cross-contamination in the dental office
   a. Gloves that are torn or punctured should be discarded and replaced
   b. Gloves worn for treatment or for examination must be changed between patients
   c. sterile surgical gloves are recommended for periodontal and oral surgical procedures
   d. *Always wash hands thoroughly with antimicrobial soap before and after removal of gloves*
   e. Jewelry—rings should not be worn under gloves

C. **Contaminated personal protective equipment must be placed in an appropriate designated area or container for washing, decontaminating, or discarding**

D. **Protective barriers are used to cover surfaces and equipment such as light handles or x-ray unit heads (Figure 8–1)**
1. Plastic covers used to protect surfaces must be replaced when contaminated.
2. Surfaces not covered by protective barriers must be cleaned and surface disinfected with an approved EPA intermediate-level disinfectant

E. **High-volume oral evacuation system minimizes the formation of aerosol during patient treatment**
1. Pre-procedural rinse and pre-brushing is recommended for patient prior to treatment to minimize bacterial counts and reduce aerosol contamination
2. Use of a rubber dam for clinical procedures reduces aerosol contamination

Personal Protective Equipment

Disposable face mask
Disposable gloves
Face shield
Protective eyewear
Clinic jackets/lab coats

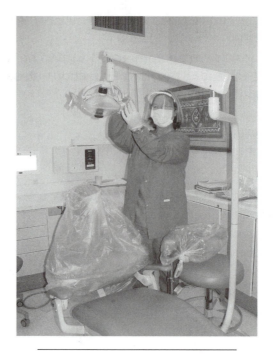

FIGURE 8–1. Personal protective equipment and barriers.

VI. HANDWASHING

A. Before placing gloves hands should be washed thoroughly with a liquid antimicrobial soap

B. Surgical procedures require the use of a standard surgical scrub; hands, wrists, and arms up to the elbow are scrubbed with overlapping circular strokes and sufficient soap lather

VII. STERILIZATION

A. **Sterilization** destroys all forms of microscopic life, including bacterial spores and viruses by chemical or physical agents

   1. Methods of sterilization

      a. Steam under pressure—moist heat

      b. Chemical vapor

      c. Dry heat

      d. Ethylene oxide

      e. High-level disinfectant for items that cannot endure heat

   2. Sterilization equipment is considered a medical device and is regulated by the U.S. Food and Drug Administration (FDA)

B. **Asepsis** is a term used to describe freedom from pathologic microorganisms (**pathogens**); conversely, **sepsis** refers to the existence of disease-producing microorganisms

C. All instruments that will penetrate soft tissue or come in contact with bone must be sterilized

   1. Centers for Disease Control and Prevention recommends identifying items according to the way in which an instrument contacts patients

---

Methods of Sterilization

Dry heat
Steam autoclave
Chemical vapor
Ethylene oxide
High-level disinfectant

2. Spaulding modified classification system
    a. Critical—instruments that penetrate soft tissue or bone
    b. Semi-critical—instruments that touch oral tissues but do not penetrate soft tissues must be sterilized after each use
    c. Non-critical—instruments that will not be used in the mouth but will come in contact with intact skin

D. Packaging materials—sterilization method compatibility
1. Steam under pressure—autoclave (250 to 275°F) pouches, paper/plastic, paper, nylon, polypropylene
2. Chemical vapor (250°F)—pouches, paper/plastic, paper
3. Dry heat (320°F)—pouches, paper/plastic, paper, nylon closed containers
4. Packaging materials are considered Class II devices and must be cleared by the U.S. Food and Drug Administration
5. Tape or heat-seal pouches according to manufacturer's recommendation
6. Label in pencil and date package

E. Chemical vapor sterilizers use agents such as formaldehyde, alcohol mixtures (Figure 8–2)
1. Use of chemical vapor sterilizers requires adequate ventilation because of the release of potentially harmful vapors
2. Sterilizer effective for carbon steel instruments

F. Dry heat method of sterilization is effective for instruments that tend to rust or dull easily; cycle is 1 hour in length
G. Immersion method of chemical sterilization
1. High-level disinfectant must be EPA-approved and registered as a "sterilant/disinfectant"
2. Exposure cycle for immersion method of chemical sterilization may be as long as 10 hours

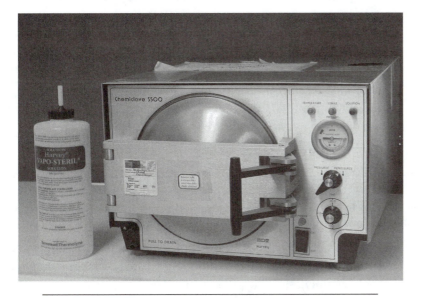

FIGURE 8–2. Chemical vapor sterilizer.

Sterilization Monitoring Methods

Biological monitoring (spore testing)
Chemical monitoring
Physical monitoring

Biological Monitoring (Spore Testing)

Positive test results indicate sterilization failure
Negative test results indicate sterilization

H. Ethylene oxide sterilization methods are used for plastic, cloth, rubber masks, and nitrous oxide rubber hoses, cycle averages a minimum of 12 hours

VIII. **STERILIZATION MONITORING**

A. Weekly monitoring of dental sterilizers is recommended by the Centers for Disease Control and Prevention (CDC)

B. **Biological monitoring (spore testing) provides the best means of verification for assurance of sterilization**
   1. Biologic indicators are placed inside the chamber during processing in the center of the load
   2. Biologic indicator contains bacterial endospores used for spore testing
   3. Biological indicator may be housed in self-contained spore vials, or paper spore strips in protective glassine envelopes
   4. At the end of the cycle the biologic indicator is removed and incubated to determine if the bacterial spores were killed
   5. A control biological indicator is *not* run through the sterilization cycle
   6. The control is incubated and analyzed to confirm that if live spores are present they can yield growth
   7. *Positive* biological indicator test indicates sterilization failure; *negative* biological indicator test indicates sterilization

C. Biological indicators
   1. Bacillus stearothermophilus spores for steam and chemical vapor sterilizers
   2. Bacillus subtilis spores for dry heat and ethylene oxide sterilizers

D. Biological indicator systems
   1. In-office method requires, vials, incubator, and log book
   2. Mail-in service through FDA registered facility with culturing lab

E. Physical monitoring is performed by observing the gauges or dials on the sterilizers and recording the sterilizing temperature, pressure, and exposure time

F. Chemical change indicators are used on the outside of an instrument pack/pouch, autoclave tape, paper strips, labels
   1. Color changes occur with the chemical sensors once exposed to heat and pressure
   2. Indicators identify that the instruments have been heat processed but does not assure sterilization

Levels of Disinfection

Low-level disinfection is used for general housekeeping
Intermediate-level disinfection must display "tuberculocidal" and "hospital disinfectant" label
High-level disinfection kills spores

IX. **DISINFECTION**

A. Disinfection destroys most microorganisms by either physical or chemical agents

B. Three levels of disinfection are classified according to the biocidal activity of the product
   1. Low-level disinfection is used for general housekeeping procedures
   2. **Intermediate-level disinfection** must display a label indicating "**tuberculocidal**," "hospital disinfectant"
   3. **High-level disinfection** is capable of killing spores (**sporicidal**)

C. Following manufacturer's directions for contact time designates whether the disinfectant is used for disinfection or as a sterilant

D. Disinfectants are used on environmental surfaces (counter tops) and other inanimate fixtures such as the dental unit and dental chair

E. Disinfectant chemical agents may cause eye irritation and toxicity from inhaled fumes; adequate ventilation is required; chemical agents commonly used in the dental office include:
   1. Glutaraldehydes
   2. Sodiom hypochlorite
   3. Iodophors
   4. Synthetic phenol compounds
   5. Chemical germicide registered with the EPA as a hospital disinfectant

F. When using disinfectants note expiration dates and follow manufacturer's directions

X. DENTAL LABORATORY DISINFECTION

A. Chemical disinfectants are used in the dental laboratory to disinfect contaminated impressions, dental prostheses, and wax bites

B. To prevent damage to impressions, follow manufacturer's recommendations for appropriate use of disinfectant agents when performing **decontamination** procedures

C. All items that have been used in the mouth carry the potential for cross-contamination

D. If an impression or contaminated item has not been disinfected and sent to the dental laboratory it must be placed in a leak proof sealed bag and identified with a biohazard label

XI. PRE-TREATMENT INFECTION CONTROL

A. Pre-treatment infection control requires pre-cleaning before spraying with an intermediate-level disinfectant

B. Flush dental unit retraction valve water lines for at least one minute prior to the beginning of each clinic day; water lines are also flushed after treatment of each patient

C. During the dental procedure, a separate disposable bag should be used to dispose of contaminated soiled materials such as bloody gauze or cotton rolls

XII. POST-TREATMENT INFECTION CONTROL

A. Heavy utility gloves are used to wipe down contaminated environmental surfaces and when handling soiled instruments

B. Surfaces must be clean of any debris or bioburden in order for a disinfectant to be effective

---

When Using Disinfectants

Use manufacturer's recommended dilutions for concentrated agents

Clean instruments prior to immersion in high-level disinfectant

Follow proper exposure time cycles

Store and handle according to specifications

Do not use on certain metals or vinyl materials

Check expiration dates

Provide adequate ventilation

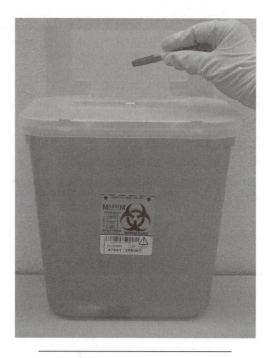

FIGURE 8–3. Sharps container.

C. Regulated medical waste is to be discarded in a separate plastic bag indicated for that purpose

1. Disposable needles and other sharp disposable items must be disposed of in a puncture-resistant, leakproof container (Figure 8–3)
2. Biohazard symbol must be affixed to the container

XIII. PREPARING DENTAL INSTRUMENTS FOR STERILIZATION

A. Steps for sterilizing instruments

1. *Transport* contaminated instruments to the processing area carefully to prevent exposure and injury from sharp items
2. *Cleaning* of bioburden by utilizing an ultrasonic cleaner or instrument washer

---

Steps for Sterilizing Instruments

1. Preclean—holding solution
2. Clean—ultrasonic unit
3. Packaging—packs, trays, cassettes
4. Sterilization—heat sterilization
5. Storage—store in aseptic area

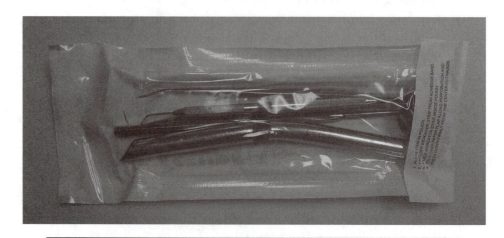

FIGURE 8–4. Packaging of loose instruments.

3. *Packaging* of loose instruments (Figure 8–4)
   a. Select appropriate packaging for method of sterilization and place chemical indicator inside pack
   b. Follow manufacturers instructions for sealing package
   c. Packages are dated on the date processed in pencil
4. *Sterilization* load sterilizer according to the manufacturer's instructions; Allow packs to dry and cool before handling (Figure 8–5)
5. *Storage* of sterilized packs and instruments must be in a clean dry environment
6. *Delivery* of packs in manner that maintains integrity and sterility of instruments until ready for use

B. Quality assurance incorporates record keeping, equipment maintenance, and biologic monitoring results

XIV. RADIATION ASEPSIS

A. Basic infection control procedures must be initiated when exposing and processing radiographs
B. Processed x-ray films which are not in protective barrier envelopes are considered contaminated upon removal from the patient's mouth

XV. MANAGEMENT OF OFFICE WASTE

A. Regulations regarding waste management disposal must be followed according to federal, state, and local requirements
B. Medical waste is identified by using red leakproof plastic bags and the biohazard symbol, which indicate hazardous waste (Figure 8–6)
C. Dental offices may use approved waste haulers which meet EPA standards

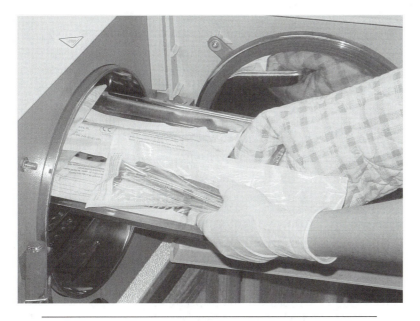

FIGURE 8–5. Loading the sterilizer.

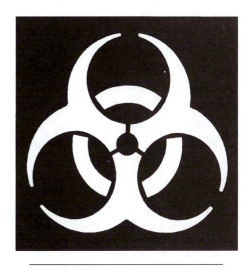

FIGURE 8–6. Biohazard symbol.

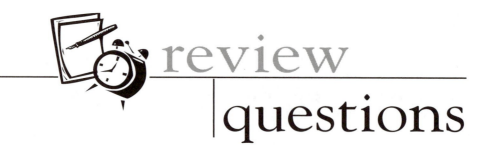
DIRECTIONS Each of the questions or incomplete statements below is followed by suggested answers or completions. Select the **one answer** that is best in each case.

1. The most effective way to kill microbes is
   A. low-level disinfectants.
   B. ultraviolet light.
   C. autoclaving.
   D. ultrasonic immersion.

2. Bactericidal refers to
   A. bacterial growth.
   B. bacteria in the bloodstream.
   C. killing bacteria.
   D. hand soaps and lotions.

3. Protective equipment and personal protection for the dental assistant who comes in direct or indirect contact with a patient's blood and saliva include all of the following EXCEPT
   A. immunization against hepatitis B.
   B. puncture proof secondary containers.
   C. facemask, gloves, protective eyewear.
   D. disposable gown.

4. A patient's medical and dental history should be reviewed
   A. before rendering clinical dental care.
   B. prior to submitting insurance forms.
   C. periodically at the recall (recare) visit.
   D. only if a surgical procedure is indicated.

5. After packaging instruments for sterilization the autoclave should be loaded
   A. slowly to prevent damage to the instrument packs.
   B. by placing instrument packs in an upright position.
   C. with as many instrument packs as possible.
   D. with both wrapped as well as unwrapped instrument packs.

6. A disadvantage of the chemical vapor sterilizer is
   A. instruments become tarnished and rusted.
   B. instruments become too hot.
   C. instruments must be carbide.
   D. adequate ventilation is required.

7. Asepsis is defined as the
   A. method for disease transmission.
   B. presence of disease producing micro-organisms.
   C. process to prevent the transmission of disease.
   D. infection which can spread.

8. Biological indicators used to test steam sterilizers contain
   A. *Bacillus stearothermophilus.*
   B. *Mycobacterium tuberculosis.*
   C. active viruses.
   D. *Streptococcus mutans.*

9. Approved intermediate level surface disinfectants may be used to clean
   A. critical instruments.
   B. environmental surfaces—walls, floors.
   C. removable appliances.
   D. waterline biofilm.

10. Hands should be washed before and after gloving with a (an)
    A. bleach and water solution.
    B. isopropyl alcohol wipe.
    C. antimicrobial hand soap.
    D. hard bristle scrub brush.

11. Disposable needles and glass anesthetic cartridges are discarded in a
    A. red biohazard puncture-proof container.
    B. standard garbage bin.
    C. plastic trash bag.
    D. sterilization pouch.

12. When handling contaminated instruments the assistant must wear
    A. examination gloves.
    B. disposable food-handler gloves.
    C. sterile surgical gloves.
    D. heavy utility gloves.

13. Dental handpieces (both high and low speed) must be sterilized
    A. once a day.
    B. after each patient.
    C. before and after lubrication.
    D. after working on a patient with a known communicable disease.

14. Ethylene oxide is a form of gas sterilization that requires approximately _____ hours for sterilization.
    A. 1 to 2
    B. 8
    C. 10 to 16
    D. 48

15. According to the Occupational Safety Health Administration (OSHA), an occupational exposure is defined as a(an)
    A. radiographic image.
    B. occupational emergency.
    C. eyewash station.
    D. contact with blood or saliva.

16. Which of the following are considered regulated waste?
    1. blood-soaked gauze.
    2. tissue samples from a biopsy.
    3. contaminated infectious disposable materials.
    4. extracted teeth.
    A. 1, 3
    B. 2, 4
    C. 3 only
    D. 4 only
    E. All of the above

17. OSHA requires employee-training programs for dental personnel
    A. once a year.
    B. who are newly hired.
    C. when they return from a vacation.
    D. prior to receiving required immunizations for hepatitis B.

18. Hazardous materials utilized in the dental office must be
    A. labeled properly with a biohazard warning symbol.
    B. labeled and identified in three different languages.
    C. stored in the refrigerator.
    D. stored in a locked file cabinet.

19. Steam under pressure/autoclaving is best suited for
    A. paper or plastic products.
    B. nitrous oxide rubber hoses.
    C. noncorrosive metal instruments.
    D. handpieces.

20. Flushing dental unit waterlines is recommended
    A. for 30 minutes at the end of the workday.
    B. between patients if a transmissible disease exists.
    C. for 30 minutes at the beginning of the workday.
    D. at the beginning of the work day and in between patients.

☑answers

rationales

1.

C. Autoclaving, steam under pressure, is the most effective way to kill microbes. The heat from the steam sterilizes the instruments.

2.

C. Bactericidal refers to killing bacteria. Bacteriostatic refers to inhibiting bacterial growth. Bacteremia is the presence of bacteria in the bloodstream.

3.

B. The OSHA category for identifying personal protective equipment (PPE) includes gloves, face mask, protective eyewear, and outerwear such as disposable gowns. Personal protection for the healthcare worker includes immunizations against hepatitis B. Secondary containers must be labeled according to OSHA standards.

4.

A. Health history questionnaires must be completed before rendering clinical dental care. A patient's medical history can affect all phases of a patient's treatment, including prescriptions, pre-operative and post-operative instructions and length of appointments.

5.

B. Instrument packs should be loaded in the sterilizer in an upright position to allow for adequate circulation of steam and heat under pressure in the chamber.

6.

D. A disadvantage of the chemical vapor sterilizer is that adequate ventilation must be provided to avoid inhalation of the chemical vapor gases released by the unit.

7.

C. Asepsis provides an environment which reduces cross-contamination and prevents the transmission of disease.

8.

A. Biologic indicators used to test steam sterilizers contain *Bacillus stearothermophilus*. The indicators contain non-disease causing spores and may also be used to test chemical vapor sterilizers.

9.

B. Approved intermediate-level surface disinfectants may be used to clean environmental surfaces such as counter tops, chairs, wall, floors. Waterline biofilm is cleaned by improving the quality of the incoming water such as filtered or purified water.

10.

C. Handwashing with an antimicrobial hand soap or solution is recommended to reduce the numbers of pathogenic microbes found on the hands and under the fingernails.

11.

A. Red puncture-proof and leak-proof containers labeled with a biohazard symbol are used to discard sharps such as scalpel blades, glass anesthetic cartridges, disposable needles and ortho wires. The sharps container should be located close to the area of operation.

12.
D. When handling contaminated instruments the assistant must wear heavy utility gloves. Heavy utility gloves are puncture resistant and assist in preventing accidental injury. A long-handled scrub brush is recommended for scrubbing instruments if an ultrasonic cleaner is not available.

13.
B. After treating each patient the high-speed and low-speed handpiece must be sterilized.

14.
C. Ethylene oxide sterilization requires approximately 10 to 16 hours for sterilization. This form of gas sterilization is an ADA-accepted form of sterilization and is most often used in hospitals. Adequate ventilation is required when utilized.

15.
D. An occupational exposure as defined by the Occupational Safety Health Administration (OSHA) include a contact made with blood, saliva, or other potentially infectious materials.

16.
E. Regulated waste includes blood-soaked gauze, tissue samples from a biopsy, extracted teeth, and contaminated infectious disposable materials.

17.
B. The Occupational Safety Health Administration (OSHA) requires employee training programs for newly hired dental personnel who may come in contact with bloodborne pathogens, saliva, or other potentially infectious materials. Dental personnel whose job descriptions change and are at risk for coming in contact with potentially infectious materials should also be trained. The employer is required to maintain records of all training.

18.
A. Hazardous materials utilized in the dental office must be labeled properly with a biohazard warning symbol and/or a chemical warning label providing information regarding the hazards of the chemical contents of the product. Warning information may include steps for proper storage and handling. Labels must be written legibly and prominently displayed.

19.
C. Steam under pressure/autoclaving (moist heat sterilization) is best suited for noncorrosive metal instruments.

20.
D. Flushing dental unit waterlines is recommended at the beginning of the work day and between patients. Recommended flushing times vary from 3 to 5 minutes at the start of the day and 20 to 30 seconds between patients.

9

Occupational Safety

contents

➤ Bloodborne Pathogen Standard

➤ Controlling Occupational Exposure

➤ Engineering and Work Practice Controls

➤ Housekeeping

➤ Waste Handling

➤ Recordkeeping — Medical and Training Records

➤ Hepatitis B Vaccination

➤ Laundry

➤ Exposure Control Plan

➤ Exposure Incident Follow-Up

➤ Employee Communication Program

➤ Hazard Communication Standard

➤ Material Safety Data Sheets

➤ Labeling

➤ Training and Employee Information

➤ Written Hazard Communication Program

➤ Dental Office General Safety and Product Safety Guidelines

The Occupational Safety and Health Administration (OSHA), a division of the United States Department of Labor, is the regulatory body which oversees the protection of all workers from physical, chemical, or infectious hazards in the workplace. This chapter will present an overview of the OSHA Bloodborne Pathogen Standard and Hazard Communication Standard.

KEY TERMS

Bloodborne pathogen standard

Biohazard

Engineering controls

Exposure incident

Eyewash station

Hazard communication standard

Hepatitis B virus

Human immunodeficiency virus

Material safety data sheet

Office safety program coordinator

OSHA

Source individual

Work practice controls

Written exposure control plan

Written hazard communication program

OSHA Requirements: Occupational Exposure to Bloodborne Pathogen Standard

1. Personal protective equipment
2. Engineering work practice controls
3. Housekeeping
4. Waste handling
5. Employee medical records/vaccination
6. Laundering
7. Written exposure control plan

Personal Protective Equipment

Face shield/face mask
Eyewear
Clinic jacket/lab coat
Disposable gloves
Utility gloves
Resuscitation bags/mouthpieces

I. BLOODBORNE PATHOGEN STANDARD

A. **Bloodborne pathogen standard** was initiated to provide protection to all healthcare workers who come in contact with bloodborne pathogens

B. Bloodborne pathogens can exist in blood or other body fluids such as saliva
   1. **Hepatitis B virus** (HBV)
   2. **Human immunodeficiency virus** (HIV)

C. Components of **OSHA**'s bloodborne pathogen standard
   1. Personal protective equipment (PPE)
   2. Establishment of engineering/work practice controls
   3. Housekeeping
   4. Waste handling
   5. Employee medical records/vaccination records
   6. Laundering
   7. Written exposure control plan

II. CONTROLLING OCCUPATIONAL EXPOSURE TO BLOODBORNE PATHOGENS (Figure 9–1)

A. Occupational exposure refers to reasonably anticipated skin, eye, mucous membrane, or parenteral contact with blood

B. Healthcare workers must not allow blood or other potentially infectious materials (OPIM) to pass through to clothing, skin, or mucous membranes

C. Personal protective equipment for dental healthcare workers refers to barriers that are worn to protect the worker from bloodborne pathogens, OPIM, and hazardous materials
   1. Face mask—mask must be worn under face shield
   2. Eyewear—goggles or eyeglasses with side shields

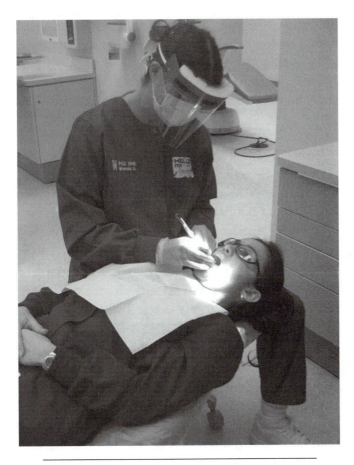

FIGURE 9–1.   Controlling exposure to pathogens.

3. Clinic jackets/lab coats
4. Gloves
5. Ventilation devices/resuscitation bags, mouthpieces, pocket masks

D. Contaminated nondisposable clinic wear must be placed in an appropriate designated area for washing and decontaminating

III. ENGINEERING AND WORK PRACTICE CONTROLS

A. Engineering controls include special containers for contaminated sharp instruments
1. Engineering controls isolate or remove the hazard from employees
2. Rubber dams, high-speed evacuators, and sharps containers are examples of engineering controls
3. Employers must consider safer needle devices when conducting a review of the annual exposure control plan with team members, methods for evaluating new devices that will reduce exposure are identified

B. Work practice controls alter the manner in which a task is performed to reduce the likelihood of exposure
1. Wash hands immediately after skin contact with blood or other potentially infectious materials
2. Flush mucous membranes immediately if they are splashed with blood or other potentially infectious materials

---

Engineering Controls

Engineering controls isolate or remove the hazard from the employee (e.g., rubber dam, sharps container)

Work Practice Controls

Work practice controls alter the manner in which the task is performed (e.g., prohibiting bending of contaminated needles)

3. Eliminate the bending or breaking of contaminated needles

4. Recapping of needles by using mechanical device or one-handed scoop technique

5. Discard contaminated needles in sharps container that is puncture resistant, leakproof, colored red, and marked with a **biohazard** symbol

6. Eating, drinking, smoking, applying cosmetics, and handling contact lenses in areas where there is occupational exposure is prohibited

7. Eliminate the storage of food and drink in refrigerators, cabinets, shelves, or countertops where blood or OPIM are present

8. Contaminated extracted teeth, tissue, and or impressions, if transported, must be placed in closed containers that are leakproof, colored red and affixed with a biohazard symbol

IV. HOUSEKEEPING—All surfaces, equipment, and other reusable items must be decontaminated with a disinfectant when contamination occurs through splashes, spills, or other contact with blood or OPIM

V. WASTE HANDLING

A. Waste removed from the facility may be regulated by a combination of local, state, and federal laws

B. Contaminated disposable sharps must be placed in containers that are closable, puncture resistant, leakproof, colored red, and labeled with a biohazard symbol (Figures 9–2 & 9–3)

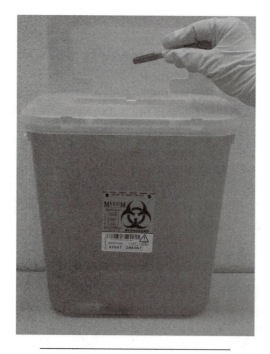

FIGURE 9–2.   Sharps container.

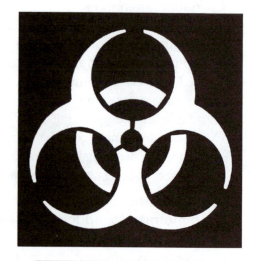

FIGURE 9–3.   Biohazard symbol.

C. Regulated waste is defined as liquid or semi-liquid blood or other potentially infectious materials; items contaminated with blood or OPIM that would release these substances in a liquid or semi-liquid state if compressed

D. Items that are caked with dried blood or OPIM and are capable of releasing these materials during handling, contaminated sharps; and pathological and microbiological wastes containing blood or OPIM are also considered regulated waste

VI. RECORDKEEPING—medical and training records

A. Medical records must be established for each employee with occupational exposure, records are confidential

  1. Records contain the hepatitis B vaccination status
  2. Occupational exposure incidents and testing results
  3. Medical records must be kept 30 years past the last date of employment of the employee

B. Training records must be kept by the employer for three years

  1. Training records document dates of training, the trainer's name and qualifications
  2. If the employer ceases to do business, medical and training records are transferred to the successor employer

VII. HEPATITIS B VACCINATION—must be made available to every employee within 10 working days of initial assignment

VIII. LAUNDRY

A. Contaminated laundry should be handled as little as possible with minimum agitation

B. Laundry that is sent off-site for cleaning must be in bags or containers that are clearly marked with the biohazard symbol

IX. EXPOSURE CONTROL PLAN

A. **Written exposure control plan** must include identification of job classifications and tasks

B. Written exposure control plan must be accessible to employees and updated at least annually, employers under the revised OSHA Bloodborne Pathogens Standard (Needlestick Safety and Prevention Act, 2001) obligate employers to consider safer needle devices when they conduct an annual review of their exposure control plan with employees

C. Provides a schedule of how and when the provisions of the standard will be implemented including schedules and methods for communication of hazards to employees

D. Provides procedures for evaluating the circumstances of an **exposure incident** and includes provisions designed to maintain privacy of employees who have experienced needle sticks

X. EXPOSURE INCIDENT FOLLOW-UP

A. Exposure incident is a specific eye, mouth, other mucous membrane, non-intact skin, or parenteral contact with blood or OPIM that results from the performance of an employee's duties

1. Puncture from a contaminated sharp instrument is an example
2. Contact to skin or eyes use copious amounts of water to area or seek **eyewash station**

B. Employees should immediately report exposure incident to the employer

1. Report initiates the procedure for request for evaluation of "source individual"
2. **Source individual** is any patient whose blood or body fluids are the source of an exposure incident to the employee
3. The results of the source individual's blood tests are confidential
4. Test results of the source individual's blood must be made available to the exposed employee through consultation with the healthcare professional

C. Employer must provide the attending healthcare professional with the following information:

1. Bloodborne pathogens standard
2. Description of employee's job duties relative to the incident
3. Incident report
4. Route(s) of exposure
5. Source individual's blood test results if available
6. Employee medical records/vaccination status
   a. Baseline blood test to establish the employee's HBV and HIV status will be drawn if employee consents (Figures 9–4 & 9–5)
   b. Employee has a right to decline testing or to delay HIV testing for 90 days
   c. Attending healthcare professional must preserve the employee's blood sample

D. Following post-exposure evaluation, the healthcare professional will provide a written opinion to the employer

1. Written opinion is limited to a statement that the employee has been informed of the results of the evaluation, and told of the need, if any, for further evaluation or treatment
2. All other findings are confidential

XI. EMPLOYEE COMMUNICATION PROGRAM

A. Training for dental employees regarding the bloodborne pathogen standard must be provided at no cost to the employee and during working hours

B. The **office safety program coordinator** must communicate the following information

1. Copy of bloodborne pathogen standard and explanation of content
2. Epidemiology and symptoms of bloodborne diseases
3. Modes of transmission of bloodborne pathogens
4. Written exposure control plan

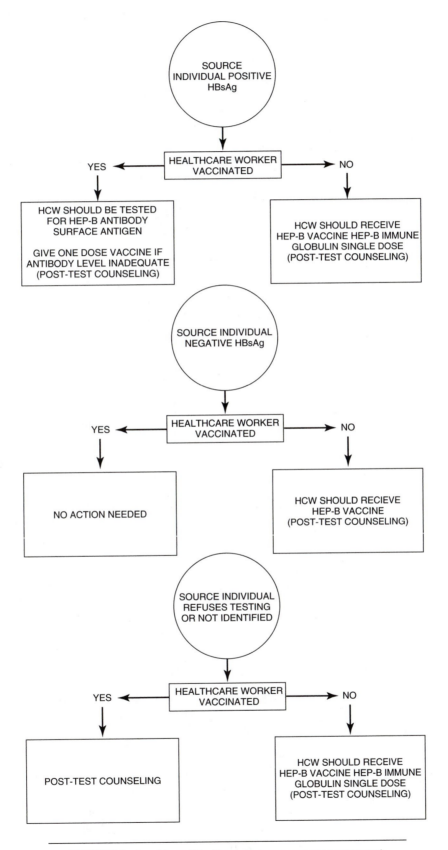

FIGURE 9–4. Hepatitis B post-exposure management.

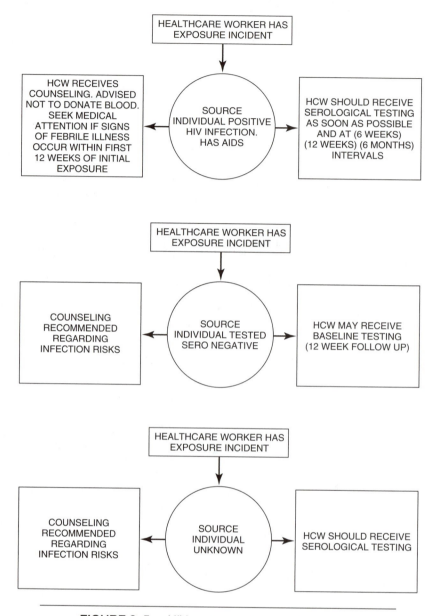

FIGURE 9–5. HIV post-exposure management.

5. How to recognize an occupational exposure
6. Methods to control occupational transmission of bloodborne pathogens
7. Personal protective equipment
8. Hepatitis B vaccine and vaccination information
9. Emergencies involving blood and OPIM
10. Reporting mechanisms for exposure incidents
11. Post-exposure evaluation and follow-up
12. Explanation of labels, signs, markings for contaminated materials
13. Discussion of preventive measures including engineering and safe work practice controls, housekeeping, universal precautions
14. Allow for questions and answers

XII. HAZARD COMMUNICATION STANDARD

A. **Hazard communication standard** was initiated to protect all workers who may come in contact with potential injuries and illnesses from exposure to hazardous chemicals in the workplace
   1. Includes physical hazards such as flammability
   2. Includes health hazards such as irritation, lung damage

B. **Requirements of Hazard Communication Standard**
   1. Material Safety Data Sheets (MSDS)
   2. Labeling
   3. Record keeping
   4. Written Hazard Communication Program

XIII. MATERIAL SAFETY DATA SHEETS (Figure 9–6)

A. Chemical manufacturers and importers must develop a **material safety data sheet (MSDS)** for each hazardous chemical they produce or import
   1. MSDS must be in English
   2. Identify chemical and include common name
   3. Known acute and chronic health effects of chemical
   4. Exposure limits
   5. Whether the chemical is considered to be a carcinogen
   6. Precautionary measures
   7. Emergency and first-aid procedures
   8. Identification of the organization responsible for preparing the material safety data sheet

B. **Employers must prepare a list of all hazardous chemicals in the workplace**
   1. Copies of the MSDS for hazardous chemicals are to be readily accessible to employees in that area
   2. MSDS sheets may be kept in a binder in a central location or accessed by computer terminals

XIV. LABELING (Figure 9–7)

A. Chemical manufacturers, importers, and distributors must label, tag, or mark all containers of hazardous chemicals

B. In the workplace, the employer is responsible for labeling secondary containers which contain hazardous chemicals such as ultrasonic units, x-ray wet tanks containing developer and fixer solutions
   1. Secondary container must show hazard warnings appropriate for employee protection
   2. Hazard warning can be any type of message, words, pictures, or symbols that convey the hazards of the chemical(s)
   3. Labels must be legible, in English (other language if desired) and prominently displayed
   4. Office labeling must be easy to read and employees must be properly trained to clearly understand the system
   5. If blank containers are used labels may be photocopied from original container
   6. Labels may be color-coded for ease in identification

Hazard Communication Standard

1. Material Safety Data Sheets (MSDS)
2. Labeling
3. Record keeping
4. Written Hazard Communication Program

MATERIAL SAFETY DATA SHEET

SECTION I - MATERIAL IDENTIFICATION AND USE

Controlled Product Yes ☐ No ☑

Material Name: Ultra-Etch® 35% and 10%	Product Identification Number: REF/UP 163, 164, 167, 168, 271, 272, 273, 274, 677, and 685.
Manufacturer's Name: Ultradent Products, Inc.	Chemical Family: Acids
Street Address: 505 West 10200 South	Chemical Formula: 35% - H₃PO₄

Chemical Formula: $35\% - H_3PO_4$

City: South Jordan   State: Utah   USA

$10\% - H_3PO_4$

Zip: 84095   Emergency Telephone No. 800-552-5512

Trade Name and Synonyms: Ultra-Etch® - Enamel and Dentin Etch

Chemical Name: Phosphoric Acid

Material Use: Etching of tooth enamel and dentin.

Molecular Weight: N/A

SECTION II - HAZARDOUS INGREDIENTS OF MATERIAL

Hazardous Ingredients	Approximate Concentration %	C.A.S. N.A. or U.N. Numbers	"Exposure limits"	LD₅₀/LC₅₀ Specify Species and Route
Phosphoric Acid	35%	7664-38-2		LD₅₀ - oral rat 1530 mg/kg
Phosphoric Acid	10%	7664-38-2		LD₅₀ - oral rat 1530 mg/kg

SECTION III - PHYSICAL DATA FOR MATERIAL

Physical State: Gas ☐ Gel ☑ Solid ☐

Odor and Appearance: Odorless; Blue (35%), Bright Red (10%)

Odor Threshold (p.p.m.): N/A

Specific Gravity: 1.32 (35%) / 1.12 (10%)

Vapor Pressure (mm Hg): N/A   Vapor Density (Air = 1): N/A   Evaporation Rate: N/A

Boiling Point (°C): about 100°C

Freezing Point (°C): about -1°C

Solubility in Water (20° C): 95%   % Volatile (by volume): N/A   pH: < 2

Coefficient of water/oil distribution: N/A

SECTION IV - FIRE AND EXPLOSION HAZARD OF MATERIAL

Flammability: Yes ☐ No ☑   If Yes, under which conditions:

Means of Extinction: N/A

Special Procedures: N/A

Flash point (°C) and Method: N/A   Upper explosion limit (% by volume): N/A   Lower explosion limit (% by volume): N/A

Auto Ignition Temperature (°C): N/A   Hazardous Combustion Products: N/A

Explosion Data Sensitivity to Mechanical Impact: N/A   Rate of Burning: N/A   Explosive Power: N/A   Sensitivity to Static Discharge: N/A

SECTION V - REACTIVITY DATA

Chemical Stability: Yes ☑ No ☐   If No, under which conditions:

Incompatibility to other substances: Yes ☑ No ☐   If Yes, which ones: Bases (strong), common metals.

Reactivity and under what conditions: Chemical reaction when mixed together with bases, corrosive.

Hazardous Decomposition Products: Oxides of phosphorus.

Material Name/Identifier: Ultra-Etch

ULTRADENT PRODUCTS, INC.

FIGURE 9–6. Material safety data sheet (MSDS). (Courtesy of Ultradent Products, Inc.)

SECTION VI - TOXICOLOGICAL PROPERTIES OF PRODUCT

Route of Entry	☑ Skin Contact	☐ Skin Absorption	☑ Eye Contact	☐ Inhalation Acute	☐ Inhalation Chronic	☑ Ingestion

Effects of Acute Exposure to Product

Skin - may cause skin irritation. Eyes - severe eye irritaion. Ingestion - possible irritation.

Effects of Chronic Exposure to Product Skin - mild irritation. Eyes - damage eyes (chronic exposure must be avoided). Ingestion - irritation will occur.

LD$_{50}$ of Product (Specify Species and Route)	Not established.	Irritancy of Product	Mild	Exposure limits of Product	N/A
LC$_{50}$ of Product (Specify Species)	N/A	Sensitization to Product	N/A	Synergistic materials	N/A

☐ Carcinogenicity   ☐ Reproductive effects   ☐ Teratogenicity   ☐ Mutagenicity   N/A

SECTION VII - PREVENTIVE MEASURES

Personal Protective Equipment Protective Eyewear

Gloves (Specify)	Rubber	Respiratory (Specify)	N/A	Eye (Specify)	Protective Plastic.	Footwear (Specify)	N/A
Clothing (Specify)	N/A	Other (Specify)	N/A				

Engineering Controls (e.g. ventilation, enclosed process, specify) N/A

Leak and Spill Procedure Clean up with wet rag. Neutralize with baking soda.

Waste Disposal Wipe up and throw in trash.

Handling Procedures and Equipment Use gloves and protective eyewear.

Storage Requirements Store at room temperature.

Special Shipping Information None

SECTION VIII - FIRST AID MEASURES

Skin Flush with water.

Eye Flush immediately with water. Get medical attention.

Inhalation N/A

Ingestion Do not induce vomiting. Give large amounts of water or milk. Take an antacid. Call physician.

General advice FOR DENTAL USE ONLY - Use as directed.

SECTION IX - PREPARATION DATE OF M.S.D.S.

Additional Information Only very small dosages are used in dentistry - usually not hazardous.

Sources Used Raw Material MSDS and MFG's Knowledge.

Prepared by:	John Tobler, Chemist	Phone Number	800-552-5512	Date	September 7, 1995

The information and recommendations are taken from sources believed to be accurate; however, Ultradent Products, Inc., makes no warranty with respect to the accuracy of the information or the suitability of the recommendation and assumes no liability to any user thereof. Each user should review these recommendations in the specific context of the intended use and determine whether they are appropriate.

#10995   R003/020796

ULTRADENT PRODUCTS, INC.

FIGURE 9–6.   (Continued)

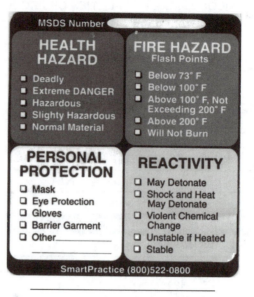

FIGURE 9–7. Labeling sample. (Courtesy of Smart Practice.)

XV. TRAINING AND EMPLOYEE INFORMATION

A. Each employee who may by exposed to hazardous chemicals must be provided information and training prior to initial assignment

B. Exposure or "exposed" under the OSHA standard means that an employee is subjected to a hazardous chemical in the course of employment

1. Routes of entry inhalation, ingestion, skin contact or absorption
2. Includes potential accidental or possible exposure

C. Information regarding hazards and protective measures is provided to workers through written labels and material safety data sheets

XVI. WRITTEN HAZARD COMMUNICATION PROGRAM

A. Workplaces where employees are exposed to hazardous chemicals must have a **written hazard communication program**

B. The employer is responsible for the development, implementation, and maintenance of the written hazard communication program

1. Prepare an inventory of chemicals
2. Ensure containers are labeled and describe labeling method
3. Obtain MSDS for each chemical and determine how list will be kept current
4. Make MSDS available to workers
5. Conduct training of workers, include how to use MSDS
6. Identify coordinator of office program
7. Maintain a description of the procedure used to train employees
8. Maintain details of the protective measures used to protect employees
9. Plan emergency exposure incident reporting and follow-up procedures

---

Written Hazard Communication Program

1. Prepare inventory of chemicals.
2. Ensure containers are labeled.
3. Obtain MSDS for each chemical. Keep current.
4. Make MSDS available to employees.
5. Conduct training of how to use MSDS.
6. Identify who is delegated to coordinate office Haz. Mat. standard.
7. Training descriptions.
8. Protective measures used to protect employees.
9. Emergency exposure incident reporting.

XVII. DENTAL OFFICE GENERAL SAFETY AND PRODUCT SAFETY GUIDELINES

A. Dental office general safety guidelines

1. Properly discard chemicals which are no longer used or have expired
2. Use protective equipment to minimize chemical contact to skin and hands
3. Provide proper ventilation to minimize inhalation of chemicals and use respiratory protection and NIOSH-approved masks
4. If chemicals contact the eye, flush with cold water and seek medical attention as soon as possible
5. Neutralizing agents such as baking soda are effective for certain acid spills
6. First-aid kit, portable oxygen resuscitation equipment, and fire extinguisher are essential in promoting general dental office safety
7. Use eye protection when working with acid etchants, if eye contact occurs, flush with cold water, maintain temperature-regulated eye-wash station (Figure 9–8)
8. Use a mask when working with alginate powders
9. Gloves and eye protection are recommended when working with disinfectants
10. Always wear gloves when working with mercury
11. Well-ventilated area is required when working with nitrous oxide gas
12. Hazardous chemicals such as acetic acid and hydroquinone are found in radiographic film processing fixer and developer solutions
13. Protective tinted eyewear is recommended when working with light-cured restorative materials

B. Dental office product safety guidelines

1. **Acid etchants**
   a. Use eye protection
   b. Dental procedures utilize phosphoric acid in sealants, composite resins, and prior to placement of orthodontic brackets

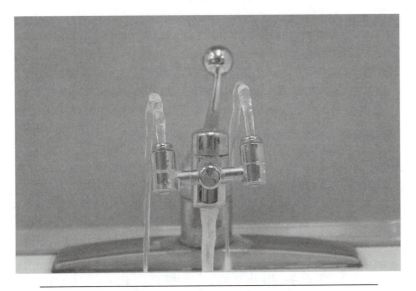

FIGURE 9–8. Eyewash station.

2. **Acidulated fluoride**
   a. Use eye protection and gloves when handling
   b. Contains small amounts phosphoric acid
   c. If eye contact flush with cold water and seek medical attention
3. **Alginate impression material**
   a. Contains silica
   b. Use a mask, protective eyewear and appropriate PPE
4. **BIS-GMA**
   a. Found in dentin bonding systems and composite resins
   b. Irritant to skin and eyes
   c. Avoid prolonged exposure; wear gloves to clean spills
5. **Bonding agents for porcelain**
   a. Used for porcelain repair or bonding agent
   b. If skin contact remove contaminated clothing and flush affected area with water, then wash soap and water
   c. Sweep up spills and place absorbent materials in container
6. **Dental stone**
   a. Contains 100% gypsum
   b. Particles may become airborne use protective eyewear and mask
7. **Disinfectant**
   a. Potent and considered hazardous
   b. Use PPE, proper ventilation is recommended
   c. If eye contact flush with water and seek medical attention
   d. Spills may be soaked up with absorbent materials and placed in a container for disposal
8. **Formaldehyde**
   a. Used in chemical vapor sterilization
   b. Eye and skin irritant use appropriate PPE
   c. Toxic by inhalation keep area well-ventilated and if spill mop up with wet mop
9. **Glass ionomer cement**
   a. Liquid/powder dental material
   b. Liquid contains polycarboxylic acid an eye and skin irritant
   c. Use appropriate PPE and in case of spills mop up liquid with wet mop and sweep powder
10. **Mercury**
    a. Gloves should be worn when handling mercury
    b. Source of contamination may be through inhalation of mercury vapor
    c. If spill occurs, ventilate area and use a filter to remove mercury vapors from the air; do not use high-volume evacuation system
    d. Use a commercially available mercury spill kit
    e. Store scrap amalgam under water in sealed container
    f. Signs of excessive exposure to mercury include, weakness, fatigue, loss of appetite, tremors of the fingers, and eyelids, memory loss, depression, insomnia, dark pigmentation of the marginal gingival, allergic manifestations, and convulsions

11. **Nitrous oxide**
    a. Work in well-ventilated area
    b. Use a scavenging system in the dental operatory
    c. Store nitrous oxide tanks securely and away from heat or other flammable gases
    d. Monitor equipment on a regular basis and check for leaks in hoses, masks, and tanks
    e. NIOSH maximum exposure level of ambient gases is 25 ppm
12. **Polyether/polysulfide impression material**
    a. Use of gloves and appropriate PPE
    b. Work in well ventilated area
    c. If skin contact wash affected area with soap and water
    d. Wipe spills up with cloth or sponge and dispose of in a closed container
13. **Radiographic chemicals**
    a. Gloves and eye protection are recommended when working with chemicals such as acetic acid and hydroquinone found in radiographic film processing fixer and developer solutions
    b. If eye contact flush eyes with cold water for at least 15 minutes and seek medical attention
    c. If skin contact remove contaminated clothing and wash affected area with soap and water
    d. Spills should be covered with baking soda and cleaned up with absorbent materials that are disposed of in a closed container
    e. Irritation to the nose and throat from vapors may also occur
    f. Work in well-ventilated area
14. **White visible light-cured materials**
    a. Wear protective tinted eyewear
    b. Potential damage to the retina of the eye may occur
    c. Avoid looking directly at the light during clinical application

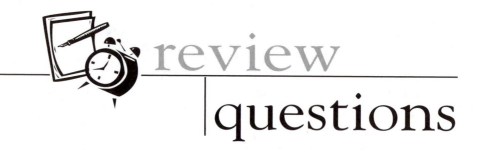

review | questions

1. The dental assistant must utilize which of the following personal protective equipment (PPE) when exposing x-ray films?
   A. lead-lined apron
   B. gloves
   C. tinted lenses
   D. moisture-proof fast film

2. Under the Occupational Safety Health Administration (OSHA) standard, the records of an employee's exposure incident are to be
   A. entered into the computer employee data file.
   B. faxed to the employee's physician.
   C. kept on file for 1 full year.
   D. kept confidential and filed in the employee's medical record.

3. When working with a visible light-cure unit
   A. the dental unit light must be turned to the off position.
   B. a face shield must be worn in place of a face mask.
   C. protective visible light eyewear is required.
   D. protective eyewear is not necessary.

4. Every dental office is required to maintain a written hazard communication program, which contains all of the following EXCEPT
   A. material safety data sheets (MSDS).
   B. laundry pick-up and delivery schedules.
   C. hazardous chemicals log.
   D. employee training records for the hazard communication standard.

5. If an immunized dental health worker experiences a percutaneous injury from a patient who is HBsAG (hepatitis B surface antigen) negative, the exposed healthcare worker should
   A. not need further treatment once immunized.
   B. begin the hepatitis series as quickly as possible.
   C. test for antibody to hepatitis B surface antigen.
   D. request that the patient see a physician as quickly as possible.

6. If a caustic chemical comes in contact with the eyes, which of the following steps must be taken?
   A. File an exposure incident report then rush to hospital.
   B. Close eyes and apply tinted protective eyewear.
   C. Flush eyes with cool water from nearest eyewash station.
   D. Flush eyes with hot, sterile water from dental unit.

7. Labeling of hazardous products in the dental office is required if the hazardous product
   A. has a shelf life.
   B. must be refrigerated.
   C. is a prescription drug.
   D. is transferred to a secondary container.

8. OSHA guidelines require employers to establish a written exposure control plan that includes
   A. engineering and work practice controls.
   B. identification of job classifications and salary scale.
   C. information on airborne particles and contaminants.
   D. employee's medical records.

9. The best way to recap a needle is to
   1. throw the needle away in the trash can.
   2. use a needle recapping device.
   3. bend the needle then remove with needle holder.
   4. utilize the one handed scoop technique.
   A. 1, 2
   B. 1, 3
   C. 1, 2, 3
   D. 4 only
   E. 2, 4

10. OSHA standards regarding contaminated laundry include all of the following EXCEPT
    A. a washer and dryer may be used on site.
    B. employee training is not required.
    C. it must be handled as little as possible.
    D. laundry transport bags must be identified with a biohazard symbol.

11. Housekeeping responsibilities of the dental assistant include decontamination of semicritical items such as
    A. dental instruments and surgical trays.
    B. dental patient chairs and units.
    C. high and low speed handpieces.
    D. dental charts and x-rays.

12. Regulated waste is identified as
    A. flammable materials.
    B. soiled laundry.
    C. disposables and uncapped needles.
    D. blood soaked gauze, saliva, and infectious materials.

13. The OSHA Hazard Communication Standard provides the employee with information regarding all of the following EXCEPT
    A. fire safety and clean-up procedures for acid spills.
    B. ventilation requirements for chemical vapor sterilization.
    C. training sessions for safe handling of hazardous chemicals including radiographic processing chemicals.
    D. education regarding the benefits of vaccinations.

14. Personal protective equipment (PPE) may include
    A. gloves, eyewear, and surgical gowns.
    B. oxygen and nitrous masks.
    C. mouthguards.
    D. long-sleeve disposable gloves.

15. OSHA's Bloodborne Pathogen Standard pertains to all employees who may come in contact with
    1. blood.
    2. saliva.
    3. other potentially infectious materials (OPIM).
    4. x-rays.
    A. 1 only
    B. 2, 4
    C. 1, 2, 3
    D. 4 only
    E. All of the above

16. Methods of reducing hazards in the dental office include all of the following EXCEPT
    A. washing hands before and after removing gloves.
    B. supplying a functional fire extinguisher.
    C. keeping the office well ventilated.
    D. playing soft music and speaking slowly to patients.

17. Vaccination of employees against the hepatitis B virus must be provided by the dentist within
    A. 1 week of employment.
    B. 10 days of employment.
    C. 1 month of employment.
    D. 1 year of employment.

18. Containers used for transport of regulated waste must be labeled with a
    A. red biohazard symbol.
    B. black poison control label.

C. material safety data sheet.

D. green chemical reactivity sticker.

19. According to OSHA guidelines employee training records relative to the Bloodborne and Hazard Communication Standard must be maintained for a minimum of

A. 6 months.

B. 1 year.

C. 3 years.

D. 30 years.

20. Biologic monitoring is perfomed when sterilizing instruments with

    1. heat-sensitive indicator tape.

    2. sealed glass ampules containing non-pathogenic spores.

    3. color-coded autoclave bags.

    4. test strips impregnated with non-pathogenic spores.

A. 1, 3

B. 2, 4

C. 1, 2, 3

D. 4 only

E. All of the above

answers & rationales

1.

B. If handling contaminated exposed x-ray film the dental assistant must wear gloves. Personal protective equipment (PPE) by OSHA standards includes; gloves, face mask, eyewear, and protective outerwear which is long-sleeved and high-necked.

2.

D. The records of an employee's exposure incident are to be kept in a confidential employee medical record file. The employer is responsible for the file, which must be retained for the duration of an employee's employment plus 30 years.

3.

C. Protective visible light eyewear is required to protect the eyes from retinal damage.

4.

B. Laundry delivery schedules and the office costs for laundry service are not part of the OSHA written hazard communication program.

5.

A. If a dental healthcare worker is immunized for hepatitis B and is exposed through a percutaneous injury to a source individual who has tested HbsAG (hepatitis B surface antigen) negative no further treatment or vaccinations are necessary for the healthcare worker.

6.

C. If a caustic substance comes in contact with the eyes, flush the eyes immediately at a temperature regulated eyewash station or with fresh running water and seek medical attention as quickly as possible. The employee must report exposure incidents in the workplace to the employer.

7.

D. Labeling of hazardous products is required if the product is transferred to a secondary container. Labeling provides important information regarding directions for product use, disposal, storage, and personal protective requirements when handling. X-ray tanks containing developer and fixer solutions are examples of secondary containers that require labeling.

8.

A. Exposure control plans must include engineering and work practice controls which assist in removing the potential hazard from the employee and alter the manner in which a task is performed. Information on job classifications and identification of task risks and exposure incident reporting procedures are also required in the exposure control plan.

9.

E. The best way to recap a needle is to use a needle recapping device or the one-handed scoop technique to prevent an accidental needle stick (occupational exposure).

10.

B. Employee training is required regarding the steps for handling, transporting, and/or decontaminating soiled laundry.

11.

B. Housekeeping responsibilities of the dental assistant include decontamination of work surface areas and equipment contaminated by splashes, spills or other potentially infectious materials.

12.

D. Regulated waste is defined as liquid or semi-liquid blood or other potentially infectious materials that would release these substances in a liquid or semi-liquid state if compressed; contaminated sharps, and pathological and microbiological wastes containing blood or other potentially infectious materials.

13.

D. The OSHA Hazard Communication Standard provides the employee with information and training regarding the potential dangers associated with hazardous chemicals and products in the dental office. Fire safety and information on disposal and clean-up procedures for hazardous chemicals are included in this standard. The OSHA Bloodborne Pathogen Standard protects the employee from transmission of bloodborne diseases such as HIV and HBV.

14.

A. Personal protective equipment (PPE) includes disposable gloves, protective eyewear, disposable face mask, and surgical scrubs or disposable protective clinical outer-apparel.

15.

C. To be in compliance with OSHA guidelines, members of the dental team who may come in contact with blood, saliva, or other potentially infectious materials (OPIM) must wear personal protective equipment and employ universal (precautions) standards when treating all patients.

16.

D. Dental assistants may reduce the potential for occupational hazards in the workplace by wearing appropriate PPE and performing proper hand-washing techniques before and after gloving to prevent cross-contamination. Fire-safety protocols should be practiced routinely including maintaining a functional fire extinguisher. A well-ventilated office reduces the potential of occupational exposure to inhalation of hazardous chemicals.

17.

B. Vaccination of employees against the hepatitis B virus must be provided by the dental employer within 10 days of the employee's start date of employment. The cost of the vaccination must be incurred by the employer. If an employee declines the vaccination documentation of the declination must be kept on file.

18.

A. Containers used to transport regulated waste must be identified with a red biohazard label. Items which are identified as being a biohazard are often placed in red bags or red containers, which are puncture resistant and, leakproof.

19.

C. Employee training records relative to the Bloodborne and Hazard Communication Standard must be maintained for a minimum of 3 years. Training records must be made easily accessible for employees to review and copy upon request.

20.

B Monitoring office sterilizers at least once a week with biologic indicators are Centers for Disease Control and Prevention (CDC) guidelines that many states now mandate. Biologic monitoring systems are available in sealed glass ampules and biological indicator test strips impregnated with nonpathogenic spores. A sterilization biological monitoring log must be maintained by the office safety coordinator.

CHAPTER

10

Medical Emergencies

contents

➤ Medical History

➤ Vital Signs

➤ Office Preparation for an Emergency

➤ Emergency Kit and Equipment

➤ Respiratory Emergencies

➤ Artificial Respiration

➤ Cardiovascular Emergency

➤ Shock

➤ Postural Hypotension

➤ Cerebrovascular Accident

➤ Convulsive Disorders

➤ Choking

➤ Metabolic Disorders

➤ Bleeding Disorders

➤ Drug-Induced Emergencies

This chapter provides a synopsis of several specific medical emergencies, including clinical patient signs and symptoms. An overview of related medical emergency procedures and office protocol is given, including medical emergency equipment, supplies, medications, and patient vital signs.

KEY TERMS

Allergy	Pulse rate
Anxiety	Shock
Cardiopulmonary resuscitation (CPR)	Sphygmomanometer
Convulsion	Syncope
Cyanosis	Systolic
Diastolic	Trendelenburg position
Hyperventilation	Vasodilator
Hypotension	

I. MEDICAL HISTORY—Must be updated and reviewed before administering direct patient clinical care

A. The best way to treat an emergency is to prevent its occurrence

1. Collect information about patient's medical and dental history; inform office personnel of patient's needs and potential emergency situation
2. Note patient information about:
   a. Drug **allergies** (hypersensitivity)
   b. Prophylactic antibiotic coverage
   c. History of infectious disease
   d. Diseases with related oral manifestations
   e. Physiologic changes such as pregnancy
   f. Psychologic disorders

B. Illnesses currently under treatment by a physician that may contraindicate certain dental procedures must be noted (Table 10–1)

1. Include name and telephone number of the patient's personal physician
2. Document information clearly in patient's dental chart

II. VITAL SIGNS

A. Critical life-saving information may be obtained by taking and recording the patient's vital signs

B. Vital signs include blood pressure, pulse rate, respiration rate, and body temperature

C. Blood pressure (Figure 10–1)

1. Blood pressure is measured during systole, the contraction phase of the heart
2. Recorded as the **systolic** blood pressure measurement

Vital Signs

Blood pressure
 Systolic
 Diastolic
Pulse rate
 60–100 per minute
 Radial artery pulse point
Respiration rate
 16–20 per minute
Body temperature
 98.6°F or 37°C

TABLE 10-1   MEDICAL PREVENTIVE REVIEW

AIDS	Consult with patient's physician regarding current health status. Patient may be immunocompromised (selective dental treatment). Antibiotic premedication may be required. Transmittable disease.
Alcohol/Substance Abuse	Possible liver dysfunction. Increase risk of prolonged clinical duration anesthetics. Increase risk heart valvular damage (antibiotic premedication required). Avoid products containing alcohol.
Arthritis/Rheumatism	Possible blood clotting disorder if on long-term medications, antiinflammatory agents, aspirin (salicylates). Corticosteroid therapy long-term requires special precautions.
Cancer	Consult with patient's physician regarding current health status. Patient may be on CNS depressants. If immunocompromised selective dental treatment is recommended. Antibiotic premedication may be required due to decreased resistance to infection.
Blood Dyscrasias	All bleeding disorders must be evaluated prior to dental treatment.
Emphysema	May require supplemental oxygen therapy during dental treatment due to reduced respiratory reserve. Nitrous-oxide is contraindicated.
Heart Valve Prosthesis	Recommendation for antibiotic premedication prior to dental treatment. Parenteral prophylactic antibiotic required for extensive surgical dental procedures.
Hepatitis	Liver dysfunction. Cautious use of dental anesthetics to avoid overdosage. Clinical duration of anesthetic action is prolonged. Consult with physician.
Kidney Problems	May require antibiotic premedication in chronic cases. Consult with physician prior to dental treatment.
Rheumatic Fever/ Congenital Heart Disease	Consult with patient regarding history rheumatic fever and affects of rheumatic heart disease. Antibiotic premedication required to minimize risk of sub-acute endocarditis (SBE).
Tuberculosis	Consult regarding disease status-active/arrested. Transmittable disease. Avoid use of aerosols, cavitron, air-jet polishers. If active disease status use disposable inhalation sedation equipment.
Ulcer	Note anxiety levels of patient. Patient may be unable to tolerate additional stress from dental treatment. Medications prescribed include tranquilizers and antacids.
Venereal Disease	Observe extraoral and intraoral tissues for oral lesions. If open weeping lesions defer dental treatment and reschedule patient.

3. During the relaxation phase, diastole, the **diastolic** blood pressure value, is measured
4. Blood pressure is measured as a fraction (e.g., 120/80)
   a. The 120 indicates the systolic pressure reading
   b. The 80 indicates the diastolic pressure reading
5. Blood pressure is measured with an aneroid **sphygmomanometer**
6. Stethoscope is used to listen to the Korotkoff sounds produced by the **brachial artery** altered blood flow from pressure of sphygmomanometer cuff
7. Hypertension indicates elevated high systolic or diastolic arterial blood pressure value
8. **Hypotension** indicates low diastolic arterial blood pessure value

D. **Pulse rate is most frequently felt at the *radial artery* pulse site located on the thumb side of the wrist (Figure 10–2)**
   1. Average pulse rate for adult males is 60 to 100 heartbeats per minute
   2. Women and children tend to have slightly higher pulse rates
   3. During CPR the pulse rate is taken at the **carotid artery** pulse site on the side of the neck
   4. Weak or irregular pulse rates should be recognized and recorded in the patient's dental record

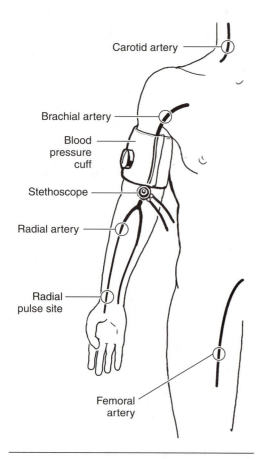

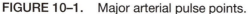

FIGURE 10–1. Major arterial pulse points.

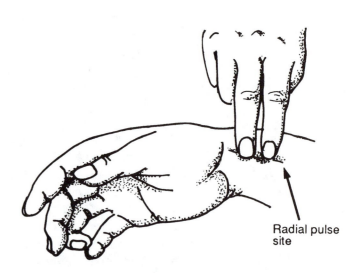

FIGURE 10–2. Position of fingers to monitor pulse.

Emergency Support
Phone Numbers

Fire department
Physician
Hospital
Pharmacy
Police department

E. Respiration rate average for adults is 16 to 20 breaths per minute
  1. Respiration is measured as one complete inspiration and exhalation of air by the lungs
  2. No movement of the chest or abdomen indicates respiratory failure; emergency steps to administer **cardiopulmonary resuscitation (CPR)** should begin immediately.
F. Body temperature average measurement is 98.6°F; elevated temperatures may indicate other serious complications

III. OFFICE PREPARATION FOR AN EMERGENCY
  A. Emergency support telephone numbers should be prepared in advance and posted in convenient locations near each office telephone
  1. Fire department
  2. Physician
  3. Hospital—emergency room extensions
  4. Pharmacy
  5. Police department
  6. Medical office if in same building

B. Emergency kit and equipment should be readily available and easy to access in the event of an emergency (Figure 10–3)

    1. Kit should include basic equipment

        a. Oxygen delivery system with barrier devices

        b. Noninjectable drugs

        c. Injectable drugs, EpiPen

        d. Equipment to monitor vital signs

        e. Airway device

        f. Tourniquets

        g. Aromatic ammonia inhalants

        h. Analgesics

        i. Anticonvulsant, diazepam

        j. Antihypoglycemic, sugar

        k. **Vasodilators,** nitroglycerin

        l. Vasopressors

IV. RESPIRATORY EMERGENCIES

A. In a respiratory emergency, a patient's breathing stops or is reduced to a level at which the body cannot support its oxygen needs

B. Respiratory failure can occur from:

    1. Airway obstruction

    2. Hyperventilation

    3. Bronchial asthma

    4. Heart failure

    5. Acute pulmonary edema

C. Respiratory emergency treatment

    1. **Hyperventilation**

        a. Sit upright

        b. Have patient breathe deeply into paper bag to increase CO_2 blood level

---

Respiratory Emergency Treatment

Hyperventilation—Sit upright and have patient breathe deeply into paper bag to build level of CO_2.

Bronchial asthma—Stop treatment, use bronchial dilator.

Heart failure—Sit upright, administer O_2, call for emergency medical support.

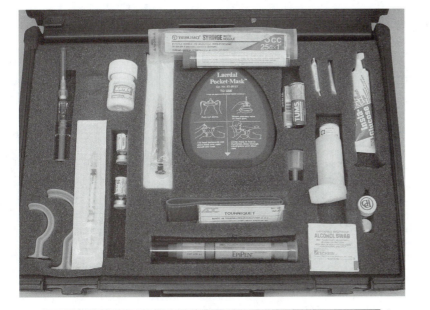

FIGURE 10–3.　Medical emergency kit.

2. Bronchial asthma
   a. Stop treatment
   b. Use bronchial dilator, oxygen, or both
   c. Cyanosis may occur in severe attack bronchial asthma
3. Heart failure and acute pulmonary edema
   a. Sit upright
   b. Administer oxygen
   c. Call for EMS—emergency medical support

Cardiopulmonary Resuscitation

CPR—Requires special training. Objective is to maintain an open airway and mechanically breathe for the victim.

V. ARTIFICIAL RESPIRATION

A. In cases of respiratory difficulty, when the heart has stopped beating, artificial respiration and CPR should be instituted

B. CPR requires special training and should be attempted only by trained individuals
1. Objective of artificial respiration is to maintain an open airway and mechanically breathe for the victim
2. Outside emergency medical assistance should be sought as quickly as possible

C. Steps in administering artificial respiration (if the patient has a pulse): mouth-to-mouth or mouth-to-mask
1. Place victim on his or her back on hard surface
2. Open airway by tipping the victim's head back until the chin is pointing upward (Figure 10–4)
3. Clear any foreign matter from the victim's mouth with finger sweep
4. Place your ear very close to the victim's mouth and look at the chest to check for breathing
5. If the victim is not breathing, pinch the nostrils closed with the fingers of the hand on the forehead, and place your mouth over the victim's mouth and deliver two slow full breaths
6. Add a breath every 5 seconds until help has arrived, the victim begins to breathe, or exhaustion overtakes you

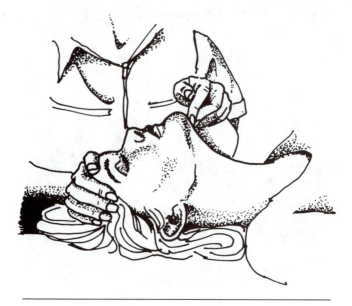

FIGURE 10–4.   Open airway by head tilt and chin lift.

7. Look, listen, and feel for breathing and check the pulse

8. If the victim begins breathing on his or her own, discontinue artificial respiration; if the victim is not breathing and has no pulse, begin chest compressions

D. Steps in administering artificial respiration (if there is severe injury to the mouth): mouth-to-nose

1. Tip the victim's head as for mouth-to-mouth resuscitation

2. Keep the victim's mouth closed by covering with your hand

3. Place your mouth over the victim's nose and blow air until the chest rises, one breath every 5 seconds

4. Place ear close to the victim's mouth (after removing your hand to allow patient to exhale air) and observe the chest to determine if the patient is breathing; look, listen, and feel

5. Add a breath every 5 seconds until help has arrived, the victim begins to breathe, or exhaustion overtakes you

6. Look, listen, and feel for breathing and check the pulse; if the victim begins breathing on his own, discontinue artificial respiration; if the victim is not breathing and has no pulse, begin chest compressions

VI. CARDIOVASCULAR EMERGENCY

A. Patients suffering from congestive heart failure (CHF) cannot lie in a supine position because of fluid retention in the lungs

B. Coronary heart disease (CHD) includes three major categories

1. Arteriosclerotic heart disease (ASHD)

2. Myocardial infarction (MI)

3. Angina pectoris

C. Myocardial infarction is caused by a sudden deficiency of oxygenated blood to the heart muscle

1. Symptoms include shortness of breath, perspiration, severe chest pain, and cyanosis

2. Make patient as comfortable as possible and relieve fear and anxiety

3. Consult with patient's physician prior to treatment for choice of anesthetic

D. Angina pectoris is a painful condition resulting from a transient deficiency of oxygenated blood supply to the heart

1. Symptoms include severe, constricting chest pain, anxiety, perspiration, and increased blood pressure

2. Administer oxygen to assist labored breathing and seat upright

3. Nitroglycerin, a fast-acting vasodilator, is given for relief of angina pectoris; nitroglycerin causes the blood vessels to relax and dilate

4. Consultation with the patient's physician is suggested before dental treatment

E. Chest pain that may or may not be caused by a cardiac emergency is managed by

1. Stopping dental treatment

2. Shifting the patient to a comfortable position

3. Administering oxygen if necessary

4. Seeking medical assistance immediately

5. Beginning basic life support if patient loses consciousness

---

Cardiovascular Emergency

CHF (congestive heart failure)—sit patient upright and seek emergency medical support.

Myocardial infarction—sit patient upright, seek emergency medical support and administer O_2.

Angina pectoris—sit upright; administer nitroglycerin sublingually.

Chest pain—discontinue treatment and seek emergency medical support.

Shock

Shock occurs when the
body's vital functions reach
a depressed state.
Anaphylactic shock—sudden
allergic reaction.
Insulin shock—hypoglycemia
or low blood sugar.

VII. SHOCK—Occurs when the body's vital functions reach a depressed state

A. **Early signs and symptoms of shock include rapid pulse, pale or cold skin, and weakness**
   1. Breathing shallow, deep and irregular, nausea, vomiting
   2. Anxiety symptoms

B. **Shock symptoms—late stage include more acute signs of unresponsiveness, eyes appear vacant with dilated pupils**
   1. Blood pressure falls and temperature decreases
   2. Loss of consciousness, death can occur

C. **Treatment for shock**
   1. Stop dental treatment
   2. Record vital signs
   3. Place patient in supine position
   4. Keep patient comfortable at room temperature
   5. Maintain airway, provide oxygen
   6. Seek medical assistance

D. **Anaphylactic shock**
   1. Anaphylaxis is a sudden allergic reaction to exposure to an allergen in the body
   2. Rapid release of histamines by the body may cause severe swelling and edema
   3. If airway becomes blocked patient may show signs of **cyanosis**, a bluish skin tone because of lack of oxygen
   4. Management of emergency requires administration of epinephrine in the arm or thigh (EpiPen)
   5. If possible administer oxygen to assist labored breathing
   6. Monitor vital signs closely
   7. Seek medical assistance

E. **Insulin shock**
   1. Diabetes is a metabolic disorder of the body
   2. Hypoglycemia when there is too much insulin in the body blood sugar is low
   3. Symptoms
      a. Headache
      b. Feelings of dizziness, vertigo
      c. General weakness,
      d. Clammy skin
      e. Confusion
   4. Management
      a. Administer something sweet to eat, sugar, candy, orange juice
      b. Consult patient's physician for follow-up treatment

F. **Diabetic coma**
   1. Patient is unconscious
   2. When there is too little insulin in the body and blood sugar is high (hyperglycemia)
   3. Seek medical assistance immediately

VIII. SYNCOPE

A. **Syncope,** or fainting, is a transient loss of consciousness that can occur during any phase of dental treatment

B. Contributing factors include **anxiety,** fear, emotional stress, exhaustion, poor physical condition

   1. Symptoms

     a. Pallor

     b. Discomfort

     c. Weakness

     d. Perspiration

     e. Cold and clammy skin

     f. Temporary loss of consciousness

   2. Treatment

     a. Place patient in **Trendelenburg position** with feet slightly elevated in relation to the head

     b. Establish airway, loosen tight clothing

     c. Spirits of ammonia

     d. Administer oxygen portable unit 100% O_2 delivery system (Figure 10–5)

IX. POSTURAL HYPOTENSION (ORTHOSTATIC HYPOTENSION)

A. Patients may experience postural hypotension if suddenly placed in an upright position

B. Symptoms

   1. Sudden drop in blood pressure

   2. Lightheadeness

Syncope

Patient will feel faint. Check vitals. Place patient in Trendelenburg position with feet elevated. Administer spirits of ammonia and O_2 if necessary.

Postural Hypotension

Caused by rapid change in body position. Place patient in supine position and administer O_2 if necessary. Monitor vital signs.

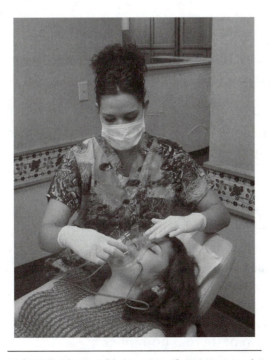

FIGURE 10–5. Placement of oxygen mask.

C. Treatment
 1. Placing the patient in a supine position
 2. Maintaining the airway
 3. Administering oxygen if necessary
 4. Slowly changing the patient's position before dismissal

Cerebrovascular Accident

CVA—Cerebrovascular accident or stroke. Seek emergency medical assistance. Monitor vital signs, administer CPR if necessary.

X. CEREBROVASCULAR ACCIDENT
 A. Stroke or cerebrovascular accident (CVA) is a neurologic disorder in the brain caused by a vascular insufficiency
 B. Signs and symptoms of major strokes
  1. Unconsciousness
  2. Paralysis or weakness of upper or lower extremities
  3. Difficulty in breathing
  4. Problem with speech
 C. Treatment for stroke requires immediate medical assistance EMS; supply life support—CPR

XI. CONVULSIVE DISORDERS
 A. Epilepsy is a chronic disease characterized by involuntary muscle contractions (**convulsions**)
  1. Mild convulsions—petit mal
  2. Severe seizures—grand mal

Convulsive Disorders

Petit mal—Mild seizures
Grand mal—Severe seizures

 B. Symptoms include muscle spasms, thrashing, drooling at the mouth, rolling eyes, and loss of consciousness
 C. Treatment of grand mal seizure includes placing patient in supine position with the head tilted to the side so that saliva and vomitus exit decreasing aspiration of fluids into lungs
  1. Loosen tight clothing
  2. Maintain an open airway
  3. Remove objects that might injure a thrashing patient
  4. Do not attempt to force any object into the patient's mouth
  5. Seek medical assistance

XII. CHOKING VICTIMS MAY BE TREATED BY ADMINISTERING ABDOMINAL THRUSTS (Figure 10–6)
 A. Place patient in a comfortable position and encourage to cough in order to remove obstruction
 B. Seek medical assistance
 C. Start basic life support if breathing stops

Diabetic Acidosis

Diabetic acidosis or hyperglycemia is caused by above normal levels of blood sugar.

XIII. METABOLIC DISORDERS
 A. Diabetes mellitus is a chronic disease associated with carbohydrate, fat, and protein metabolism
 B. Hyperglycemia as a result of above normal levels of blood sugar may present symptoms of abdominal pain, nausea, vomiting, intense thirst
  1. Acetone odor to breath
  2. Skin appears dry and flushed
  3. Seek medical assistance immediately
 C. Hyperthyroidism is a disease caused by excessive production of thyroid hormones
  1. Will cause increase in basal metabolic rate
  2. Do not administer local anesthesia with epinephrine

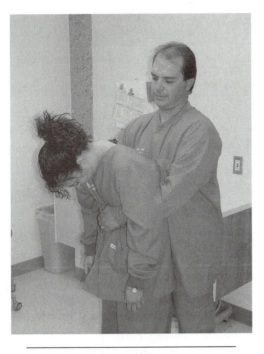

FIGURE 10–6.   Abdominal thrusts.

XIV.   **BLEEDING DISORDERS—Patients who experience clotting problems or prolonged bleeding should be closely monitored for signs of possible shock**

XV.   **DRUG-INDUCED EMERGENCIES**
   A. Complications may arise from local anesthesia; most common reaction from local anesthesia is tachycardia or rapid heartbeat
   B. Overdose of anesthetic can cause convulsive reactions or death (younger and older patients are more sensitive) (Table 10–2)
   C. Treatment for reaction to anesthetic
      1. Stop dental treatment
      2. Administer Basic Life Support (BLS)
      3. Seek medical assistance—EMS

TABLE 10–2   DOSAGE GUIDELINES FOR LOCAL ANESTHETIC AGENTS

Drug	Class	Maximum Safe Dosage
Lidocaine (Xylocaine) 2% without epinephrine	Amide	4.4 mg/kg up to 300 mg (8.3 carpules)
Lidocaine (Xylocaine) 2% with epinephrine	Amide	6.6 mg/kg up to 500 mg (13.8 carpules)
Mepivicaine (Carbocaine) 3% without vasoconstrictor	Amide	270 mg (5 carpules)
Mepivicaine (Carbocaine) 2% with 1:20,000 Neocobefrin	Amide	180 mg (5 carpules)
Prilocaine (Citanest forte) with 1:20,000 epinephrine	Amide	8 mg/kg up to 600 mg (8 carpules)
Propoxycaine (Ravocaine) 0.4% and Procaine (Novocaine) 2% with 1:30,000 levophed	Ester	The manufacturer recommends average dose of 1.8 mL although this dose may be doubled if necessary

Note: The maximum recommended dosage without significant effect at any one time is 0.2 mg which is approximately equivalent to 10 carpules of 1:100,000. Cardiac patients should always be evaluated closely with regard to the use of epinephrine. Dosage is defined as a body mass-dependent variable. Guidelines based on healthy adult male weighing approximately 70 kg.

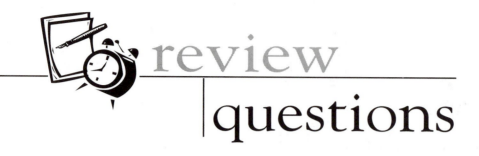

review questions

review questions

DIRECTIONS Each of the questions or incomplete statements below is followed by suggested answers or completions. Select the **one answer** that is best in each case.

1. The route of administration for drugs which enter directly into the lungs is known as
   A. intramuscular.
   B. inhalational.
   C. intravenous.
   D. intraosseous.

2. Patients who indicate on a medical history that they have rheumatoid arthritis most likely take an anti-inflammatory drug known as
   A. nitroglycerin.
   B. atropine.
   C. aspirin.
   D. amoxicillin.

3. Symptoms of cardiovascular or cerebrovascular incidents include all of the following EXCEPT
   A. weakness on one side of the body.
   B. chest pain.
   C. labored breathing.
   D. erythema.

4. Which of the following is recommended for the prevention of an asthma attack?
   A. bronchodilator
   B. ammonia vaporoles
   C. blood pressure equipment
   D. automated defibrillator

5. Medical complications for patients diagnosed with AIDS can be prevented by implementing the following procedures

   A. consulting with patient's physician prior to treatment.
   B. postponing dental treatment.
   C. minimizing aerosol production.
   D. practicing universal standards (precautions).

6. When managing a victim experiencing a grand mal seizure what treatment should be avoided?
   A. lower the dental chair and move nearby equipment to prevent injury
   B. loosen tight clothing
   C. assessment of open airway and activation of EMS(emergency medical services)
   D. forcing a mouth prop between the teeth to prevent biting the tongue

7. Antibiotic premedication is recommended for patients with a history of
   1. rheumatic heart disease.
   2. kidney dialysis/shunt placement.
   3. prosthetic cardiac valve.
   4. bacterial endocarditis.
   A. 1 and 4
   B. 1 and 3
   C. 2 and 4
   D. 4 only
   E. All of the above

8. Signs and symptoms commonly associated with insulin shock (hypoglycemia) include
   A. crushing pain in chest, slurred speech.
   B. cold sweat, weakness, dizziness.

158

C. bluish skin tone (cyanosis).

D. increased rate of respiration—hyperventilation.

9. Which of the following is the recommended method for managing air-way obstruction of a foreign body in an adult?

A. finger sweep if victim is responsive to remove object

B. abdominal thrusts (Heimlich maneuver)

C. check for breathing and pulse then begin CPR

D. place victim in supine position and begin chest compressions

10. Traumatic orofacial injuries may include all of the following EXCEPT

A. dislocated mandible.

B. avulsed tooth.

C. facial bone fracture.

D. abrasion of cervical tooth surfaces.

11. Syncope refers to

A. a sudden state of excitement.

B. spasms of the facial muscles.

C. loss of consciousness.

D. hypertension.

12. The color of the nitrous oxide cylinder tank is

A. blue.

B. green.

C. red.

D. yellow.

13. The depressed state of many body functions is called

A. shock.

B. depression.

C. epileptic.

D. toxic.

14. When taking a blood pressure reading, the first sound heard is the

A. diastolic pressure.

B. systolic pressure.

C. carotid pressure.

D. femoral pressure.

15. The administration of an excess amount of a drug is known as

A. toxemia.

B. hyperarrested.

C. actual dose.

D. overdose.

16. Symptoms of postural hypotension include

A. profuse sweating.

B. elevated high blood pressure.

C. low blood pressure.

D. a sudden state of excitement.

17. Anaphylactic shock is

A. a chronic allergic reaction.

B. the result of aspirating a foreign object.

C. an acute allergic reaction.

D. best treated with the patient in a seated position.

18. Knowledge of the patient's medical and dental history might affect

1. the treatment plan.

2. the drugs prescribed.

3. the length of the scheduled appointments.

4. the method of payment.

A. 1, 4

B. 1, 2, 3

C. 2, 4

D. 4 only

E. All of the above

19. Acetone breath, dry mouth, thirst, and weak pulse are possible symptoms of

1. hypertension.

2. epilepsy.

3. kidney disease.

4. diabetic coma.

A. 1, 3

B. 2, 4

C. 1, 2, 3

D. 4 only

E. All of the above

20. If performing CPR on a patient with a history of an infectious disease, the rescuer should always

1. wear disposable gloves.

2. not perform CPR until EMS arrives.

3. use protective devices or a microshield.

4. obtain a thorough health history first before beginning CPR.

A. 1, 3

B. 2, 4

C. 1, 2, 3

D. 4 only

E. All of the above

☑ answers & rationales

1.

B. The route of administration for drugs which enter directly into the lungs is known as inhalational.

2.

C. Aspirin is a mild analgesic that has antipyretic (fever-reducing) and anti-inflammatory properties.

3.

D. Cardiovascular emergencies involve the heart. Congestive heart failure and myocardial infarction are two examples. Symptoms may include shortness of breath, perspiration, severe chest pain and cyanosis. Cerebrovascular incidents involve a neurologic disorder in the brain caused by a vascular insufficiency. Symptoms may include weakness on one side of the body. Erythema refers to diffuse redness over the skin which may be caused by overexposure to heat, cold, or ionizing radiation.

4.

A. Respiratory drugs used to treat asthma produce a bronchodilation effect to assist breathing. Use of a bronchodilator provides a rapid release of the medication and is easy to transport.

5.

A. Medical complications for patients diagnosed with AIDS can be prevented by consulting with the patient's physician prior to treatment.

6.

D. When managing a victim experiencing a grand mal seizure it is best to avoid forcing a mouth prop between the teeth to wedge the mouth open.

7.

E. Antibiotic premedication is recommended for patients with a history of rheumatic heart disease, bacterial endocarditis, prosthetic cardiac valves, surgically constructed shunt placement and kidney dialysis. The American Heart Association standard regimen recommended is: 2 grams Amoxicillin 1 hour prior to the dental procedure. If unable to take Amoxicillin because of allergy Clindamycin may be substituted.

8.

B. Signs and symptoms commonly associated with insulin shock (hypoglycemia) include; dizziness, weakness, and a cold sweat.

9.

B. The recommended method for managing airway obstruction of a foreign body in an adult regardless of whether the victim is responsive or unresponsive includes opening of the airway with a tongue-jaw lift, look in the airway, and try to remove the foreign body with a finger sweep. If these actions are unsuccessful you then perform abdominal thrusts (Heimlich maneuver).

10.

D. Traumatic orofacial injuries do not include cervical abrasion of tooth surfaces. Cervical abrasion is often caused by incorrect toothbrushing techniques and the use of a hard bristle toothbrush and abrasive toothpaste.

11.

C. Syncope refers to the lack of blood to the brain for a short period. This is caused by dilation of blood vessels in the body and results in loss of consciousness.

12.

A. The color of the nitrous oxide cylinder tank is blue. Nitrous oxide tanks should be checked periodically to ensure that they are full and functioning properly.

13.

A. The depressed state of many body functions is called shock. The severity of shock depends on the cause. Some forms of shock are neurogenic, insulin, and anaphylactic.

14.

B. When taking a blood pressure reading, the first sound heard is recorded as the systolic pressure measurement. Systolic blood pressure is the pressure exerted on the walls of arteries when the heart contracts.

15.

D. An overdose is the term used to identify administering an excess amount of a drug.

16.

C. Postural hypotension is most likely to occur when the patient's chair position is changed too quickly. Symptoms include lightheadedness, possible loss of consciousness, and low blood pressure. Predispos-ing factors include patients taking antihypertensive medications, antidepressants, narcotics, and drugs for Parkinson's disease. To avoid postural hypotension raise the patient in the dental chair slowly from a supine position to an upright position.

17.

C. Anaphylactic shock is a sudden violent allergic reaction. Two drugs used in dentistry that may cause this reaction are local anesthesia and penicillin. A detailed accurate medical history or past adverse drug reactions could indicate whether a drug could cause this reaction.

18.

B. A patient's medical and dental history can affect all phases of a patient's treatment, including appointment and prescriptions.

19.

D. Symptoms of diabetic coma (ketoacidosis) include weak pulse, low blood pressure, dry mouth and thirst, flushed skin tone, confusion, general weakness or drowsiness, and acetone breath odor. Diabetic coma may occur from an insufficient amount of insulin or failure to take insulin medication when indicated.

20.

A. If performing CPR on a patient with a history of an infectious disease, the rescuer should wear disposable gloves and use a protective microshield or use mouth-to-mask ventilation.

Dental Practice Management

contents

➤ The Office Manual

➤ Personnel Management

➤ Telephone Communication

➤ Patient Reception

➤ Patient Records

➤ Record and Bookkeeping Systems

➤ Appointment Book and Day Sheet

➤ Recall (Recare) System

➤ Accounts Receivable and Payable Management

➤ Third-Party Carriers

➤ Inventory Systems

This chapter provides an overview of the business aspect of the professional dental practice and the role of the dental office business manager. Knowledge of accounting, recordkeeping, computer skills, third-party payment plans, patient communication skills, OSHA regulations, appointment control, collections, financial payment arrangements, inventory systems, supervisory skills and related legal aspects of dentistry as they apply to these procedures is required of the business dental assistant.

KEY TERMS

Accounts payable	Insurance carrier
Accounts receivable	Inventory
Confidentiality	Malpractice
Consultation	Negotiate
Credits	Receipt
Debits	Reconcile
Excluded	Reimburse
Facsimile (fax)	Third-party payment
Informed consent	Verification

I. THE OFFICE MANUAL

A. An office manual is a reference guide that contains detailed descriptions of all office policies and procedures
B. Office manual is utilized to facilitate training of new employees
C. Guidelines for office manual may include
   1. Doctor's philosophy of practice
   2. Job descriptions of all team members
   3. Employment policies
      a. Working hours
      b. Vacation
      c. Sick leave
      d. Overtime
      e. Holidays
      f. Dismissal
      g. Termination
      h. Bonus profit-sharing plan
   4. Office policies for the staff
      a. Dress code
      b. Conduct
      c. Staff meetings
      d. Continuing education
   5. Guidelines for appropriate office communication
      a. Telephone technique
      b. Reception policies
      c. Written correspondence
      d. Patient education

Office Manual Components

1. Office philosophy
2. Job descriptions
3. Employment policies
4. Office policies
5. Communication procedures
6. Maintenance office records
7. Clinical procedures
8. Medical emergency protocols
9. General office safety
10. Quality assurance

      6. Policies for management of office records
         a. Clinical and financial patient records
         b. Payment and collection procedures
         c. Accounts receivable
         d. Accounts payable
         e. Insurance coverage
         f. Recalls
         g. Inventory
      7. Guidelines for clinical procedures
         a. Preparation of tray setups
         b. Sterilization techniques
         c. Prescriptions
         d. Laboratory interactions
         e. OSHA regulations
      8. Medical emergency office protocol and procedures
      9. General office safety
         a. Fire safety
         b. Location of material safety data sheets (MSDS)
    10. Quality assurance policies and procedures

II. PERSONNEL MANAGEMENT

A. Written employment agreement is recommended for all new employees

B. Employment agreements are signed by the employee and employer and are usually done in duplicate

    1. Outline starting salary and range
    2. Working hours
    3. Probationary period
    4. Information regarding termination procedures
    5. Job duties
       a. State dental practice act of approved auxiliary duties under general or direct supervision of a dentist
       b. Employee evaluations and when conducted
         1) Specifications on certain work practice and engineering controls

C. Employers must comply with federal employment and hiring laws

    1. The American with Disabilities Act (ADA) applies to fair hiring practices and elimination of discrimination against individuals who are disabled
    2. Strict attention must be paid to federal laws regarding fair hiring and firing practices of all employees
    3. Title II of the American with Disabilities Act mandates access to public service by the disabled

III. TELEPHONE COMMUNICATION (Figure 11–1)

A. The telephone image conveyed by the auxiliary should encourage a friendly, trusting attitude in the caller

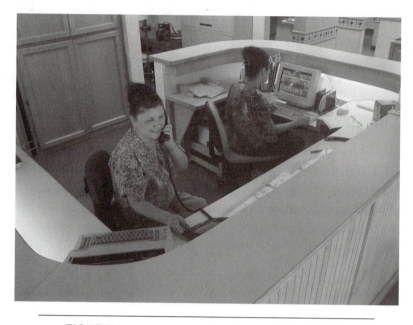

FIGURE 11–1. Front office business assistants.

B. Recorded messages on answering machines should be clear and understandable
1. Obtain name and telephone number
2. Purpose of call
3. Dental problem or concern
4. What will happen as result of call (e.g., the call will be returned)

C. Phone conversations should be conducted in a professional and courteous manner
1. If a caller is to be placed on hold ask for the caller's permission first
2. If necessary you may need to return a call and should ask the caller when it is best to return the call

D. An avulsed tooth injury requires professional emergency dental treatment
1. If providing emergency instructions by phone, primary instructions should emphasize
   a. Importance of professional emergency dental treatment
   b. Suitable transport media if unable to replant avulsed tooth into socket
   c. Transport media includes milk, saline, saliva (buccal vestibule)
2. Inform caller that the tooth should not be rinsed if placed in water
3. If the avulsed tooth can be replanted at the site of injury but is contaminated, rinse with water before replanting and seek professional emergency dental treatment

E. Voice mail systems allow incoming calls to be directed to a specific staff member

F. Facsimile (fax) machines allow written communication to be sent and received electronically through sophisticated office telephone systems

IV. PATIENT RECEPTION

A. The business assistant is the key public relations member of the office team because he or she makes the first contact with patients

B. Important patient data such as medical dental histories are often taken at the front desk reception area

C. Patient **confidentiality** should always be observed and respected

V. PATIENT RECORDS

A. Patient dental records contain confidential information
   1. Records must be filled out completely and updated periodically to avoid potential medical emergencies and legal problems
   2. **Informed consent** implies that the patient has had a thorough explanation of the required treatment and risks
   3. Obtain the patient's consent to treatment in writing provided the patient is of legal age
   4. If patient is a minor requires signature of parent or legal guardian

B. Diagnostic materials include x-ray films, information noted at the clinical examination and study models

C. Patient treatment plans must be prioritized and include a record of the total fees for services rendered

D. Before any records leave the office (e.g., for insurance purposes or **consultation** with a specialist) duplicate copies should be made for legal protection; maintain originals including radiographs; send duplicate copies
   1. Dental records are permissible evidence in a court of law
   2. All entries must be made in ink
   3. If dental records are computerized, consideration towards adequate security and confidentiality of the dental records should be given
   4. Limit number of personnel to access dental record information by issuing a password
   5. Identify authority to access, receive, or use protected health information under HIPPA

E. All office records should be protected against fire and theft

VI. RECORD AND BOOKKEEPING SYSTEMS

A. Record and bookkeeping systems encompass all paperwork pertaining to the dental practice
   1. System must be standardized and organized
   2. Provides information on past and present patient treatment
   3. Production records
   4. Precise tax information

B. Filing systems may be alphabetical or numerical

C. Patient records should never be destroyed even if deemed inactive

D. Every office should have a security alarm system to protect against theft

VII. APPOINTMENT BOOK AND DAY SHEET

A. The appointment book is the responsibility of the business assistant

B. In advance, certain periods of time should be matrixed or blocked out
   1. Elderly and young children should be scheduled early in the day when most cooperative
   2. Schedule buffer periods for unexpected emergencies

C. Broken appointments and cancellations may disrupt the schedule—create a short-notice call list to use time efficiently

D. Patients treatment may be scheduled in an appointment book or computer using time unit intervals of 10 or 15 minutes

E. Business assistant verifies that all dental laboratory casework has been returned to the office by the time of the patient's next appointment

VIII. RECALL (RECARE) SYSTEM

A. At the end of each series of treatments, the dentist or the assistant should remind the patient that they should return for an examination after a given interval of time

B. Recall (recare) methods vary and may take the form of written reminders or combination of telephone and mail notices
   1. Computer-generated record-keeping systems are used to maintain monthly recall lists
   2. Recall file cards are also maintained on a monthly basis for patient's to track their recall (recare) pattern

IX. ACCOUNTS RECEIVABLE AND ACCOUNTS PAYABLE MANAGEMENT

A. Dental practices utilize computerized bookkeeping systems or manual systems to maintain financial records
   1. Single-entry bookkeeping system records only payments
   2. Double-entry bookkeeping system records both the **debit** (charges) and **credit** (payments)
   3. Both entry systems provide the necessary information to balance the financial records and provide duplicate records

B. Daily accounts receivable bookkeeping system includes the following basic entry information:
   1. Patient name
   2. Treatment charges
   3. Payment
   4. Adjustments to the account
   5. Charge slips, encounter forms, or posting slips
   6. Receipt of the financial transaction for the day

C. Every office has a policy about payments
   1. Fees charged for services rendered represent the dentist's earnings
   2. Received payments constitute actual income
   3. For the practice to be profitable income must exceed expenses (overhead)

4. Overhead is the cost of resources needed to produce dentistry including rent, salaries, supplies, laboratory procedures
5. Expenses (overhead) of a dental practice constitute the accounts payable

D. Credit experts indicate that delinquent accounts over 90 days old are difficult and often impossible to collect

1. Business assistant has the responsibility to negotiate with the patient regarding the preferred method of payment
2. Payment methods include cash, checks, money orders, credit cards, and bank plans (Table 11–1)
3. Business assistant must monitor payment arrangements continuously
4. Financial arrangements regarding method of payment should be finalized prior to beginning treatment
5. Statements are used to remind patients of divided payment agreements
   a. Note date of expected payment
   b. Note amounts of expected payments
6. Payments not received by a specific date are to be referred to collections

E. Computerized management systems may also be employed for billing purposes and efficient process of insurance forms

1. Security issues must be considered when using computers
2. Back-up files should be created whenever possible to ensure that important information and files are not lost
3. Internal audits should be periodically monitored

F. The bank deposit slip posts an itemized list of all collected currency and received payment checks

1. Date and total amount of the deposit is clearly entered on the pre-printed office deposit slip

TABLE 11–1   PAYMENT POLICY METHODS

Method	Definition
Advanced payment	Payment before treatment is the most desirable, since billing, collection problems and accounts receivable are eliminated.
Fixed amount	The total fee is divided by the approximate number of sessions projected for completion of the treatment, and a fixed amount is expected from the patient at each visit, regardless of the actual charge for particular treatment rendered during the visit.
Divided payment	The total fee is divided into three amounts. The initial payment, usually larger than the other two, is collected when treatment commences. The balance, which is divided in half, is due when treatment is half completed and a visit or two before treatment is completed.
Open account	Patients are sent statements (forms indicating the financial status of their accounts) after treatment is rendered. This method often results in high accounts receivable, since most patients are unaware of their obligations until they receive statements, are often unprepared to pay for services rendered, or take a substantial amount of time to complete payment.

2. Duplicate copy of the completed deposit slip is kept for future reference
3. Deposits are done on a daily basis

G. **Each office may establish an office policy regarding a change fund**
   1. Change fund is the specified amount of cash used on a daily basis in the office for transactions involving change
   2. Change fund is not recorded on the bank deposit slip
   3. Petty cash fund is used for small expenses—a petty cash voucher and **receipt** for the items purchased must be maintained

H. **To reconcile (balance) a bank statement, check the number of each outstanding check and enter all debits on to the register**
   1. Verification of all deposits made should be reviewed
   2. **Debits** are considered items which have been deducted from the account
   3. Bank service charges may be included
   4. **Credits** are considered items which have been deposited into the account
   5. Credits to the account may also include earned interest
   6. Reconcile (balance) the bank statement with the checkbook as soon as the statement is received
   7. Outstanding and cancelled checks must be considered when balancing the bank statement

I. **Accurate records must be maintained according to federal regulations relative to employee's earned pay and payroll taxes**
   1. Business assistant may be responsible for preparing the payroll
   2. Each employee is required to complete an employee's withholding (W-4) form
   3. The form is a federal requirement and allows the employer to legally deduct a portion of the employee's estimated withholding tax

X. THIRD-PARTY CARRIERS
A. **The insurance carrier (insurance company that offers dental plans) is chosen by the employer for their employees**
B. **Insurance carrier agrees to cover and pay for benefits claimed under the plan (third-party payment)**
C. **Insurance companies may reimburse (repay) the doctor or the patient for dental services rendered**
   1. Amount of reimbursement may be based on usual, customary, or reasonable fees **(UCR)**
   2. **UCR** is an amount considered standard for the procedure in a given community or a fixed amount determined by the carrier for each procedure
D. **The insured patient (subscriber) should be aware of the dental insurance policy, individual benefits, and limitations**
   1. Policy deductibles
   2. Co-payments

Insurance Deductibles

An amount of eligible expenses that must be paid by the patient before the insurance plan will pay benefits

---

Insurance Co-payment

An amount paid by a health plan member for services. May be a fixed, flat fee.

3. Excluded services

4. Insurance maximum

5. Pre-treatment estimates are recommended

E. Dental patients may also maintain "dual coverage" benefits indicating that the patient has dental insurance coverage under more than one plan

1. Determine which insurance carrier is the primary carrier

2. Determine the secondary insurance carrier

3. "Birthday Rule"—used to determine which insurance carrier should be considered primary

4. Birthday rule designates that the insurance carrier for the parent who has a birthday earlier in the year is considered the primary carrier for the child

F. Specific procedure codes are established for most insurance carriers by the American Dental Association (ADA)

1. Code on Dental Procedures and Nomenclature

2. Current Dental Terminology (CDT, 4th edition) guidebook

G. Insurance claims are a form of accounts receivable

1. Insurance claims should be processed as quickly as possible

2. Electronic claims processing may be used to submit claims

H. Third-party payment plans

1. HMO—Health Maintenance Organization

2. PPO—Preferred Provider Organization

3. IPA—Independent Practice Association

4. DMO or DHMO—Dental Health Maintenance Organization

5. DRP—Direct Reimbursement Plan

XI. INVENTORY SYSTEMS

A. An inventory system is required for ordering dental supplies

1. System may be computerized

2. Tag system is used on inventory items to identify the reorder point

B. Inventory identification systems provide following information on item

1. Name of item (e.g., anesthetic)

2. Brand name (e.g., Carbocaine 2%)

3. Name of supplier, address, telephone number

4. How item is sold (e.g., box, case, package)

5. Quantity to order for the most advantageous price

6. Time at which the item should be reordered (reorder point)

7. Back orders, items previously ordered but not shipped by the supplier because of temporary unavailability

C. Storage space and location should be considered

1. X-ray film should not be stored in an area which is subject to scatter radiation, heat, or excessive light

2. Security measures—locked cabinets are required for prescription drugs stored in the office

---

Third-Party Payment Plans

HMO—Health Maintenance Organization
PPO—Preferred Provider Organization
IPA—Independent Practice Association
DHMO—Dental Health Maintenance Organization
DRP—Direct Reimbursement Plan

Inventory Identification System

1. Name of item
2. Brand name
3. Name of supplier
4. How item is sold (e.g., case)
5. Quantity to order
6. Reorder point
7. Back order log

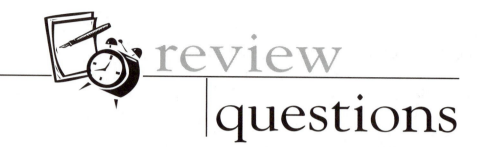

review | questions

Each of the questions or incomplete statements below is followed by suggested answers or completions. Select the **one answer** that is best in each case.

---

1. When interpreting the universal charting system for notation in a dental record
   A. teeth are numbered 1 to 32 beginning with the maxillary right third molar.
   B. teeth are numbered per quadrant from 1 through 8 beginning with third molars.
   C. teeth are lettered A through T beginning with the maxillary right second molar.
   D. teeth are numbered per quadrant from 1 through 8 beginning with central incisors.

2. A treatment plan is a (an)
   A. method of prioritizing office emergencies.
   B. system used for evaluating employees.
   C. approach to collections.
   D. systematic approach prioritizing the dental needs of the patient.

3. A running inventory is
   A. a system of altering the supply list to know which supplies are present in the office.
   B. moving the inventory from place to place.
   C. a billing technique.
   D. an inventory updated once a week.

4. Accounts receivable are
   A. monies that the dentist owes the insurance carriers.
   B. all monies owed to the dentist for completed treatment.
   C. monies that the dentist owed creditors.
   D. all monies owed to the dentist for future treatment.

5. During an office medical emergency situation the business assistant should
   1. assist the doctor and chairside assistant where needed.
   2. update the patient's health history form.
   3. call for emergency medical support personnel.
   4. administer CPR immediately to the patient.
   A. 1, 2, 3
   B. 1, 3
   C. 2, 4
   D. 3 only
   E. All of the above

6. Appointment control will
   1. prevent dental lawsuits.
   2. organize the doctor's production time.
   3. prevent emergency patients.
   4. keep hours within desired limits.
   A. 1, 2
   B. 1, 3
   C. 2, 4
   D. 3, 4
   E. All of the above

7. Responsibilities of the business assistant include all of the following EXCEPT
   A. interviewing and training new employees.
   B. maintaining OSHA employee training records.
   C. sterilizing and disinfecting instruments.
   D. entering patients in the office recall (recare) system.

8. When going through the office appointment book and blocking off time for staff meetings this procedure is known as
   A. canceling.
   B. matrixing.
   C. confirming.
   D. unit scheduling.

9. A truth-in-lending form is
   A. a contract signed by the patient.
   B. a contract signed by the doctor.
   C. a government requirement to protect all patients who pay for treatment in advance.
   D. a government requirement to protect patients from hidden finance charges in installment payments.

10. Third party refers to
    A. patients who are under the age of 18.
    B. insurance carriers.
    C. OSHA inspectors.
    D. patients receiving public assistance.

11. The period of time in which a patient may bring suit against a dentist is known as
    A. libel.
    B. malpractice time.
    C. slander.
    D. statute of limitations.

12. Mrs. Green completed her dental treatment in October. For a six-month recall (recare) she should return in
    A. April.
    B. January.

C. May.
D. March.

13. If a patient does not keep a scheduled appointment the business assistant should
    A. wait until the patient contacts the office.
    B. contact the patient as soon as possible.
    C. send the patient a statement with a charge for the broken appointment.
    D. close the patient's file and discontinue treatment.

14. When a patient calls and insists on speaking to the doctor, the assistant should
    A. call the doctor to the phone as promptly as possible.
    B. explain to the patient that the doctor will send him or her an e-mail message.
    C. explain that the doctor is treating a patient and that he or she will return the call as soon as possible.
    D. tell the patient that he or she can leave a voice mail message.

15. When a patient suffering pain of dental origin calls for an appointment, the assistant should
    A. have the patient come in immediately for temporary relief.
    B. make an appointment for next week.
    C. make an appointment the following day.
    D. refer to another dentist who is a specialist.

16. What do the letters UCR represent?
    A. unusual, coverage, receivables
    B. usual, carriers, reasonable
    C. usual, customary, reasonable
    D. usual, claims, receivables

17. Consent to an operation or to a course of treatment
    A. must be actual only.
    B. is a professional duty to the public.
    C. is not necessary for the dentist to obtain.
    D. may be expressed or implied.

18. If a patient presents inappropriate behavior while in the patient reception area, the business assistant should
    1. ask the chairside assistant to escort the patient to the dental operatory immediately.
    2. allow the patient to continue disrupting the other patients in the reception area.
    3. refer the patient to a dental specialist.
    4. speak directly to the patient in a firm but professional manner.
    A. 1
    B. 2 only
    C. 2, 3
    D. 4 only
    E. All of the above

19. An office manual is
    A. a procedural guide for all office activities.
    B. a record of Material Safety Data Sheets (MSDS).
    C. a manual describing the procedures for a dental emergency.
    D. the doctor's instructions for operating office equipment.

20. A statement of items shipped is known as a (an)
    A. cash receipt.
    B. invoice.
    C. material safety data sheet.
    D. bank statement.

1.

A. The most frequently used adult charting system is the universal numbering system, which numbers the teeth from 1 through 32, starting with the maxillary right third molar, which is numbered 1 and continuing across to the maxillary left third molar, which is numbered 16. The mandibular left third molar is numbered 17, and the numbering continues across to the mandibular right third molar, which is numbered 32.

2.

D. A treatment plan is a systematic approach to accomplishing the dental needs of the patient. This plan is made after evaluating the diagnostic materials gathered from and about the patient (e.g., medical and dental histories, radiographs, study models, clinical examination). Elements of a treatment plan include the procedure, the priority of the procedure, who will perform the task, and the amount of time the procedure requires.

3.

A. A running inventory is a system of altering the supply list to know what is present in the office. This list is updated continuously as the supplies are used. This type of system is especially important with disposable supplies.

4.

B. All treatment that has been completed and is unpaid is considered an account receivable.

5.

B. During an office medical emergency situation the business assistant should assist the doctor and chairside assistant where needed and call for medical emergency support services if indicated. Each member of the office staff should be trained in medical emergency protocol.

6.

C. Appointment control will prevent overcrowding, keep hours within desired limits, organize the dentist's production time, assign tasks to the proper individual, and provide patients with definite appointment information.

7.

C. The business assistant may often be involved in the initial or preliminary interview process and the supervision and training of new staff members in office policies and procedures. Recall (recare) system is supervised by the business assistant.

8.

B. Matrixing the appointment book designates what time periods the office is closed, such as days off, lunch time, holidays, and vacation time. Outlining the appointment book also indicates blocks of time per day that have been set aside to handle emergency appointments or staff meetings. Electronic record keeping for appointment control is also implemented in many offices.

9.

D. Any office that makes arrangements for patients to pay for their dentistry via installments is required by law to provide the patient with a truth-in-lending form. This form indicates whether or not a finance charge will be added if there is a default on payment.

10.

B. In a dental office, third party refers to an insurance carrier. All money paid by a particular insurance company is known as third-party payment.

11.

D. The statute of limitations specifies a period of time in which a patient may bring suit against a dentist. This time varies according to many factors, such as the age of the patient and the reason for the suit.

12.

A. A patient who has completed dental treatment in October and is placed on a 6-month recall will be rescheduled in April.

13.

B. It must be made very clear to all patients that the time scheduled for appointments is specifically reserved for them and that breaking appointments is unacceptable behavior.

14.

C. In an effort to conserve the doctor's time and also permit him or her to provide the appropriate attention to the patient in the chair, the business assistant should make every effort to cope with all telephone calls. In those situations wherein it is necessary for the patient to speak to the doctor, the assistant should explain that the doctor will return the call as soon as possible. It is then the assistant's responsibility to see that this promise is kept.

15.

A. When a patient suffering from pain of dental origin calls for an appointment, the dental auxiliary should obtain basic information regarding the nature of the pain, such as duration of pain, which tooth or area is involved, or if there has been a traumatic injury to the area. This basic information will assist the doctor and the chairside assistant in preparing for the emergency appointment. The patient should be given an immediate appointment for temporary relief.

16.

C. The abbreviation UCR is associated with the dental insurance fee-for-service concept. A method of calculating fee-for-service benefits is the usual, customary, and reasonable concept. *Usual* refers to the fee that the doctor charges private patients for a specific service. *Customary* fees are established if the fees fall in the same range of fees of several doctors within the same geographic area. *Customary* fees between specialists are grouped together and are considered separately from the general practitioners' fees. *Reasonable* is the concept applied to justify higher fees in cases where treatment rendered required extra time or skill due to the nature of the procedure. In these special circumstances, the doctor will increase the usual fee.

17.

D. Consent to an operation or to a course of treatment may be expressed or implied. A patient may approve of dental treatment by formally giving written consent by placing his or her signature on office consent forms or treatment plan forms. Implied consent is not as clearly defined but is interpreted by a patient's actions and behavior. When a patient offers to open his mouth for an examination, he is agreeing to treatment.

18.

D. On occasion, a disruptive patient or patients who present unusual behavior in the patient waiting room may require a firm direct approach. The auxiliary must always handle this type of situation in a professional manner. Patients suspected of substance abuse or those who are disruptive or present irrational behavior should be rescheduled.

19.

A. Every office should have a current manual that details all office tasks, policies, and procedures, in addition to goals, objectives, and philosophy of practice.

20.

B. An invoice is an itemized bill of supplies sent to the dentist. Before paying this bill, the invoice should be checked against the supplies received.

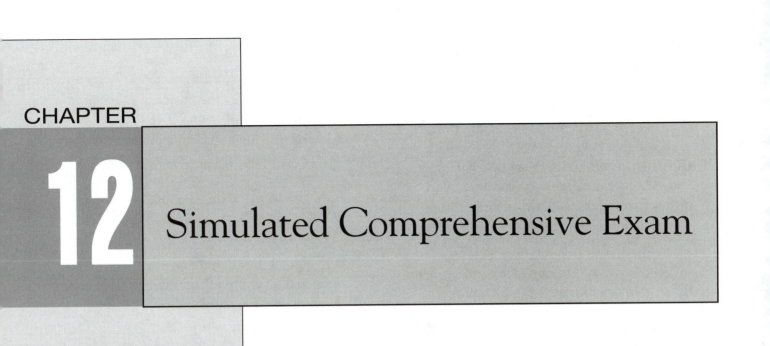

Simulated Comprehensive Exam

contents

➤ Practice Examination

➤ Answers

Each of the questions or incomplete statements below is followed by suggested answers or completions. Select the **one answer** that is best in each case.

1. When interpreting the universal charting system for notation in a dental record (Ch. 11)
   A. teeth are numbered 1 to 32 beginning with the maxillary right third molar.
   B. teeth are numbered per quadrant from 1 through 8 beginning with third molars.
   C. teeth are lettered A through T beginning with the maxillary right second molar.
   D. teeth are numbered per quadrant from 1 through 8 beginning with central incisors.

2. A treatment plan is a (an) (Ch. 11)
   A. method of prioritizing office emergencies.
   B. system used for evaluating employees.
   C. approach to collections.
   D. systematic approach prioritizing the dental needs of the patient.

3. A running inventory is (Ch. 11)
   A. a system of altering the supply list to know which supplies are present in the office.
   B. moving the inventory from place to place.
   C. a billing technique.
   D. an inventory updated once a week.

4. Accounts receivable are (Ch. 11)
   A. monies that the dentist owes the insurance carriers.
   B. all monies owed to the dentist for completed treatment.
   C. monies that the dentist owed creditors.
   D. all monies owed to the dentist for future treatment.

5. During an office medical emergency situation the business assistant should (Ch. 11)
   1. assist the doctor and chairside assistant where needed.
   2. update the patient's health history form.
   3. call for emergency medical support personnel.
   4. administer CPR immediately to the patient.
   A. 1, 2, 3
   B. 1, 3
   C. 2, 4

D. 3 only
E. All of the above

6. Responsibilities of the business assistant include all of the following EXCEPT (Ch. 11)
   A. interviewing and training new employees.
   B. maintaining OSHA employee training records.
   C. sterilizing and disinfecting instruments.
   D. entering patients in the office recall (recare) system.

7. When going through the office appointment book and blocking off time for staff meetings this procedure is known as (Ch. 11)
   A. canceling.
   B. matrixing.
   C. confirming.
   D. unit scheduling.

8. Third party refers to (Ch. 11)
   A. patients who are under the age of 18.
   B. insurance carriers.
   C. OSHA inspectors.
   D. patients receiving public assistance.

9. The period of time in which a patient may bring suit against a dentist is known as (Ch. 11)
   A. libel.
   B. malpractice time.
   C. slander.
   D. statue of limitations.

10. If a patient does not keep a scheduled appointment the business assistant should (Ch. 11)
    A. wait until the patient contacts the office.
    B. contact the patient as soon as possible.
    C. send the patient a statement with a charge for the broken appointment.
    D. close the patient's file and discontinue treatment.

11. When a patient calls and insists on speaking to the doctor, the assistant should (Ch. 11)
    A. call the doctor to the phone as promptly as possible.
    B. explain to the patient that the doctor will send them an e-mail message.

C. explain that the doctor is treating a patient and that he or she will return the call as soon as possible.
D. tell the patient that they can leave a voice mail message.

12. When a patient suffering pain of dental origin calls for an appointment, the assistant should (Ch. 11)
A. have the patient come in immediately for temporary relief.
B. make an appointment for next week.
C. make an appointment the following day.
D. refer to another dentist who is a specialist.

13. Consent to an operation or to a course of treatment (Ch. 11)
A. must be actual only.
B. is a professional duty to the public.
C. is not necessary for the dentist to obtain.
D. may be expresses or implied.

14. If a patient presents inappropriate behavior while in the patient reception area, the business assistant should (Ch. 11)
1. ask the chairside assistant to escort the patient to the dental operatory immediately.
2. allow the patient to continue disrupting the other patients in the reception area.
3. refer the patient to a dental specialist.
4. speak directly to the patient in a firm but professional manner.
A. 1
B. 2 only
C. 2, 3
D. 4 only
E. All of the above

15. A statement of items shipped is known as a (an) (Ch. 11)
A. cash receipt.
B. invoice.
C. material safety data sheet.
D. bank statement.

16. The surface of the anterior teeth facing the lips is the (Ch. 3)
A. buccal.
B. facial/labial.
C. palatal.
D. occlusal.

17. How many root canals does the maxillary first premolar have? (Ch. 3)
A. one
B. two
C. three
D. four

18. The surface of the tooth facing the midline of the mouth is the (Ch. 3)
A. mesial.
B. distal.
C. lingual.
D. incisal.

19. Congenital refers to (Ch. 2)
A. a condition at birth.
B. a condition that worsens during aging.
C. diseases of the teeth.
D. diseases of the parents.

20. The cusp of Carabelli is sometimes found on what tooth? (Ch. 3)
A. maxillary first premolar
B. maxillary second premolar
C. maxillary first molar
D. mandibular second molar

21. Exfoliation is the (Ch. 3)
A. internal absorption of succedaneous teeth.
B. removal of permanent teeth.
C. shedding of primary teeth.
D. technique used to perform a biopsy.

22. The gingival sulcus (Ch. 3)
A. lies between the free and attached gingiva.
B. is on the labial surface of anterior teeth.
C. is on the alveolar mucosa.
D. lies between the tooth and the internal surface of the free gingiva.

23. X-rays are made up of (Ch. 6)
A. electrons.
B. neutrons.
C. photons.
D. anodes.

24. Milliamperage controls (Ch. 6)
    A. the speed with which electrons move from cathode to anode.
    B. cooling of the anode.
    C. heating of the anode.
    D. heating of the cathode.

25. Collimation of the primary beam (Ch. 6)
    A. decreases the exposure time.
    B. restricts the shape and size of the beam.
    C. makes the primary beam more difficult to connect.
    D. dictates the contrast of the final radiograph.

26. The lead diaphragm determines the size and shape of (Ch. 6)
    A. electron cloud.
    B. film used.
    C. x-ray beam.
    D. filament.

27. To increase the penetrating quality of an x-ray beam, the auxiliary must (Ch. 6)
    A. increase kVp.
    B. decrease kVp.
    C. increase mA.
    D. increase FFD.

28. Filtration of the x-ray beam protects the patient by (Ch. 6)
    A. eliminating all radiation from the x-ray tubehead.
    B. eliminating weak wavelength x-rays from the x-ray beam.
    C. eliminating short wavelength x-rays from the x-ray beam.
    D. decreasing exposure time.

29. Scatter radiation is a type of (Ch. 6)
    A. secondary radiation.
    B. primary radiation.
    C. stray radiation.
    D. filtered radiation.

30. The most effective way to reduce gonadal exposure from x-rays is to (Ch. 6)
    A. increase the kVp.
    B. use a lead lined lap apron.
    C. increase vertical and horizontal angulation.
    D. use ultraspeed x-ray film.

31. The amount of radiation a person receives (Ch. 6)
    A. begins anew every day.
    B. is cumulative in the entire body.
    C. is not harmful if given in small doses.
    D. comes directly from sunlight and tanning.

32. Film speed is determined by the (Ch. 6)
    A. amount of silver bromide salts.
    B. thickness of cellulose acetate base.
    C. size of the silver bromide crystal.
    D. color of film packets.

33. The periapical film reveals (Ch. 6)
    A. the entire jaw.
    B. occlusal surfaces of upper and lower posterior teeth.
    C. lateral views of the skull.
    D. the entire tooth including the apex.

34. The principle used in panoramic radiography is (Ch. 6)
    A. long-cone paralleling principle.
    B. laminagraphy.
    C. tomography.
    D. short-cone PID's.

35. The raised button on the radiograph aids in (Ch. 6)
    A. determining the film speed.
    B. processing the film in a wet tank.
    C. identifying landmarks that are radiopaque.
    D. mounting radiographs.

36. Cone cutting results from the central ray (Ch. 6)
    A. not being aimed at the center of the film.
    B. having incorrect horizontal angulation.
    C. having increase vertical angulation.
    D. not being aimed at the intensifying screen.

37. Films not fixed for a long enough period of time will appear to (Ch. 6)
    A. have fine black lines.
    B. be clear.
    C. have a brown tint.
    D. have a thick herring bone pattern.

38. Quality assurance is necessary to ensure that (Ch. 6)
    1. x-ray film is not outdated.
    2. x-ray units are operating properly.

3. temperatures are accurate for processing.
4. test film runs are conducted periodically.
   A. 1 only
   B. 1, 3
   C. 2, 4
   D. 4 only
   E. All of the above

39. A cavity preparation that includes the mesial incisal angle of a maxillary central incisor is classified as a (Ch. 5)
   A. Class I cavity preparation.
   B. Class II cavity preparation.
   C. Class III cavity preparation.
   D. Class IV cavity preparation.

40. In application of the rubber dam, which tooth should be used as the anchor tooth? (Ch. 5)
   A. the tooth being prepared
   B. the opposing tooth being prepared
   C. one or two teeth distal to the tooth being prepared
   D. one or two teeth mesial to the tooth being prepared

41. Protective barriers are necessary when (Ch. 5)
   A. filing dental records.
   B. sterilizing instruments.
   C. reviewing a dental treatment plan.
   D. mounting x-rays.

42. During the administration of local anesthesia aspiration will (Ch. 5)
   A. damage the mandibular inferior alveolar nerve.
   B. numb the trigeminal nerve branch.
   C. determine if the lumen of the needle is in a blood vessel.
   D. cause the needle to bend.

43. The reading that is recorded first when taking blood pressure is the (Ch. 5)
   A. systolic measurement.
   B. diastolic measurement.
   C. pulse measurement.
   D. respirations per minute.

44. The assistant holds the hand instrument to be transferred between (Ch. 5)
   A. thumb and forefinger.
   B. small finger and palm.
   C. ring finger and small finger.
   D. thumb and ring finger.

45. The matrix band should be removed (Ch. 5)
   A. firmly with a serrated hemostat.
   B. quickly with a teasing motion.
   C. slowly in an occlusal or incisal direction.
   D. quickly through the sulcus.

46. Which of the following is NOT a hand cutting instrument? (Ch. 5)
   A. gingival margin trimmer
   B. hoe
   C. chisel
   D. beavertail burnisher

47. When taking an alginate impression of the upper arch the patient should be seated in a (an) (Ch. 5)
   A. slightly reclined position with the chin tilted downward.
   B. upright position with head tilted forward.
   C. upright position with head tilted back.
   D. supine position.

48. To ensure that the set alginate impression remains firmly attached in the tray during removal from the mouth the assistant should select a (Ch. 5)
   A. water-cooled tray.
   B. perforated or Rim-lock tray.
   C. compound custom-made tray.
   D. acrylic resin disposable tray.

49. A temporary filling is best packed with (Ch. 5)
   A. plastic spatula.
   B. a moist cotton pellet.
   C. a condensor.
   D. a spoon excavator.

50. Which of the following statements is true concerning placement of a wedge for a matrix? (Ch. 5)
   A. must separate the teeth slightly
   B. is used only in conjunction with the rubber dam
   C. is placed in the smallest embrasure
   D. must extend at least 3 millimeters below the gingival margin

51. Before application of a topical anesthetic the area should be (Ch. 5)
    A. examined with a explorer.
    B. dried with a 2×2 gauze square.
    C. wiped with an alcohol gauze square.
    D. dried for an x-ray exposure.

52. What instruments are best suited for removing excess cement from the teeth? (Ch. 5)
    A. low-speed handpiece with polishing cup
    B. dental floss and periodontal probe
    C. condensers and carvers
    D. explorer and scaler

53. Endodontic files are used (Ch. 5)
    A. to enlarge the root canal.
    B. to remove the contents of the pulp chamber.
    C. as drains in an endodontic abscess.
    D. to reduce the occlusal forces of an endodonticallly treated tooth.

54. A postextraction dressing can be used (Ch. 5)
    A. on a periodontal surgical site.
    B. only in impacted third molar extraction sites.
    C. if exudate is present.
    D. when there is loss of the blood clot in an extraction site.

55. On the nitrous oxide unit the flowmeter (Ch. 5)
    A. indicates the pressure of gas within the cylinder.
    B. controls the breathing bag gas reservoir flow.
    C. provides operator with a guide to the flow of volume of gas to patient.
    D. transports gas from unit to mask.

56. When applying pit and fissure sealants, it is best to (Ch. 5)
    1. use zinc phosphate cement for etching.
    2. use protective eyewear if light cured.
    3. test occlusion and interproximal contacts.
    4. apply a rubber dam or isolate with cotton rolls.
    A. 1, 4
    B. 2, 3
    C. 2, 4

D. 1, 2, 3
E. 2 only

57. When cementing temporary crowns (Ch. 5)
    1. it is best to use a temporary cement.
    2. a thick insulating base is placed in the crown prior to seating.
    3. the occlusion is checked after cementation.
    4. it is best not to use dental floss to clear the contacts.
    A. 1, 2
    B. 1, 3
    C. 2, 4
    D. 1, 2, 3
    E. All of the above

58. The mouth mirror may be used to (Ch. 5)
    1. retract the cheeks.
    2. retract the tongue.
    3. reflect light.
    4. provide indirect vision.
    A. 1, 2
    B. 1, 3
    C. 2 only
    D. 3 only
    E. All of the above

59. The dental assistant must utilize which of the following personal protective equipment (PPE) when exposing x-ray films? (Ch. 9)
    A. lead-lined apron
    B. gloves
    C. tinted lenses
    D. moisture proof fast film

60. Every dental office is required to maintain a written hazard communication program, which contains all of the following EXCEPT (Ch. 9)
    A. material safety data sheets (MSDS).
    B. laundry pick-up and delivery schedules.
    C. hazardous chemicals log.
    D. employee training records for the hazard communication standard.

61. If a caustic chemical comes in contact with the eyes, which of the following steps must be taken? (Ch. 9)

A. file an exposure incident report then rush to hospital

B. close eyes and apply tinted protective eyewear

C. flush eyes with cool water from nearest eyewash station

D. flush eyes with hot water sterile water from dental unit

62. Labeling of hazardous products in the dental office is required if the hazardous product (Ch. 9)
A. has a shelf life.
B. must be refrigerated.
C. is a prescription drug.
D. is transferred to a secondary container.

63. The best way to recap a needle is to (Ch. 9)
1. throw the needle away in the trash can.
2. use a needle-recapping device.
3. bend the needle then remove with needle holder.
4. utilize the one-handed scoop technique.
A. 1, 2
B. 1, 3
C. 1, 2, 3
D. 4 only
E. 2, 4

64. Housekeeping responsibilities of the dental assistant include decontamination of semi-critical items such as (Ch. 9)
A. dental instruments and surgical trays.
B. dental patient chairs and units.
C. high- and low-speed handpieces.
D. dental charts and x-rays.

65. Medical complications for patients diagnosed with AIDS can be prevented by implementing the following procedures? (Ch. 10)
A. consulting with patient's physician prior to treatment
B. postponing dental treatment
C. minimizing aerosol production
D. practicing universal standards (precautions)

66. OSHA's Bloodborne Pathogen Standard pertains to all employees who may come in contact with (Ch. 9)

1. blood.
2. saliva.
3. other potentially infectious materials (OPIM).
4. x-rays.
A. 1 only
B. 2, 4
C. 1, 2, 3
D. 4 only
E. All of the above

67. Methods of reducing hazards in the dental office include all of the following EXCEPT (Ch. 9)
A. washing hands before and after removing gloves.
B. supplying a functional fire extinguisher.
C. keeping the office well-ventilated.
D. playing soft music and speaking slowly to patients.

68. Vaccination of employees against the Hepatitis B virus must be provided by the dentist within (Ch. 9)
A. 1 week of employment.
B. 10 days of employment.
C. 1 month of employment.
D. 1 year of employment.

69. Containers used for transport of regulated waste must be labeled with a (Ch. 9)
A. red biohazard symbol.
B. black poison-control label.
C. material safety data sheet.
D. green chemical reactivity sticker.

70. Biologic monitoring is perfomed when sterilizing instruments with (Ch. 8)
1. heat-sensitive indicator tape.
2. sealed glass ampules containing non-pathogenic spores.
3. color-coded autoclave bags.
4. test strips impregnated with non-pathogenic spores.
A. 1, 3
B. 2, 4
C. 1, 2, 3
D. 4 only
E. All of the above

71. Calcium hydroxide is used primarily as a base to (Ch. 7)
    A. insulate the pulp thermally.
    B. insulate the pulp chemically.
    C. protect the pulp from bacteria.
    D. promote secondary dentin formation.

72. The chemical used to etch enamel is (Ch. 7)
    A. eugenol.
    B. zinc oxide.
    C. phosphoric acid.
    D. resin.

73. An impression is a (Ch. 7)
    A. negative reproduction of oral tissues.
    B. night guard mold.
    C. negative metallic casting.
    D. positive reproduction of a prepared tooth.

74. Plaster models (Ch. 7)
    A. have no dimensional change upon setting.
    B. expand upon setting.
    C. have greater crushing strength than cast stone models.
    D. are thermoplastic.

75. Acrylic resins are used for (Ch. 7)
    1. anterior restorations.
    2. temporary bridges.
    3. custom trays.
    4. temporary aluminum crowns.
    A. 1 and 4
    B. 2 and 4
    C. 1, 2, and 3
    D. 2 only
    E. All of the above

76. Characteristics of pit and fissure sealants may include (Ch. 7)
    1. self-curing polymerization.
    2. acid etching.
    3. light-cured polymerization.
    4. metallic matrix trips.
    A. 2, 4
    B. 1, 2, 3
    C. 1, 4
    D. 2 only
    E. All of the above

77. Amalgamation is the process of (Ch. 7)
    A. combining mercury with amalgam alloy.
    B. condensing amalgam into the cavity preparation.
    C. dispensing the amalgam.
    D. burnishing the amalgam against the matrix band.

78. What is the main component of composite restorative materials? (Ch. 7)
    A. polymethyl methacrylate
    B. hydrogen peroxide
    C. calcium hydroxide
    D. inorganic filler

79. A periodontal surgical pak is placed (Ch. 7)
    A. in extraction dry socket sites.
    B. around a dental implant.
    C. directly over sutures at surgical site.
    D. whenever mobile teeth are splinted.

80. Tooth bleaching is a cosmetic procedure for treating teeth with (Ch. 7)
    A. extrinsic or intrinsic stains.
    B. multiple metallic gold crowns.
    C. porcelain crowns.
    D. erosion or abrasion.

81. A frenum is a fold of mucous membrane. Frena are located (Ch. 3)
    1. in the maxillary labial vestibule.
    2. at the junction of the hard and soft palate.
    3. in the mandibular labial vestibule.
    4. at the retromolar ridge.
    A. 1 only
    B. 1 and 2
    C. 2 and 3
    D. 1 and 3
    E. 4 only

82. Which part of the tooth forms first? (Ch. 3)
    A. crown
    B. root
    C. pulp
    D. dentin

83. Each developmental lobe on molars is represented by a (Ch. 3)
    A. fissure.
    B. cusp.

C. marginal ridge.

D. groove.

84. Which of the following is recommended for the prevention of an asthma attack? (Ch. 10)
    A. bronchodilator
    B. ammonia vaporoles
    C. blood pressure equipment
    D. automated defribrillator

85. The abbreviation q4h means (Ch. 2)
    A. every four days.
    B. every four hours.
    C. take before meals.
    D. as needed.

86. Disclosing agents identify (Ch. 4)
    A. plaque.
    B. carious lesions.
    C. calculus.
    D. gingival recession.

87. A dilute sodium hypochlorite solution is recommended for cleaning (Ch. 4)
    A. partial dentures with metal clasps.
    B. full dentures.
    C. orthodontic bands.
    D. implants.

88. Calculus (tartar) has the ability to irritate the gingival tissue because it is (Ch. 4)
    1. calcified.
    2. subgingival.
    3. covered with plaque.
    4. rough and irregular in texture.
    A. 1, 4
    B. 1, 3
    C. 2, 4
    D. 3 only
    E. All of the above

89. The process of demineralization will occur with (Ch. 4)
    A. caries.
    B. calculus.
    C. green stain.
    D. yellow stain.

90. After packaging instruments for sterilization the autoclave should be loaded (Ch. 8)
    A. slowly to prevent damage to the instrument packs.
    B. by placing instrument packs in an upright position.
    C. with as many instrument packs as possible.
    D. with both wrapped as well as unwrapped instrument packs.

91. A disadvantage of the chemical vapor sterilizer is (Ch. 8)
    A. instruments become tarnished and rusted.
    B. instruments become too hot.
    C. instruments must be carbide.
    D. adequate ventilation is required.

92. Approved intermediate level surface disinfectants may be used to clean (Ch. 8)
    A. critical instruments.
    B. environmental surfaces—walls, floors.
    C. removable appliances.
    D. waterline biofilm.

93. Disposable needles and glass anesthetic cartridges are discarded in a (Ch. 8)
    A. red biohazard puncture-proof container.
    B. standard garbage bin.
    C. plastic trash bag.
    D. sterilization pouch.

94. When handling contaminated instruments the assistant must wear (Ch. 8)
    A. examination gloves.
    B. disposable food handler gloves.
    C. sterile surgical gloves.
    D. heavy utility gloves.

95. Dental handpieces both high- and low-speed must be sterilized (Ch. 8)
    A. once a day.
    B. after each patient.
    C. lubricated once a day.
    D. after working on a patient with a known communicable disease.

96. Which of the following are considered regulated waste? (Ch. 8)
    1. blood-soaked gauze
    2. tissue samples from a biopsy
    3. contaminated infectious disposable materials
    4. extracted teeth
    A. 1, 3
    B. 2, 4
    C. 3 only
    D. 4 only
    E. All of the above

97. Hazardous materials utilized in the dental office must be (Ch. 8)
    A. labeled properly with a biohazard warning symbol.
    B. labeled and identified in three different languages.
    C. stored in the refrigerator.
    D. stored in a locked file cabinet.

98. Steam under pressure/autoclaving is best suited for (Ch. 8)
    A. paper or plastic products.
    B. nitrous oxide rubber hoses.
    C. noncorrosive metal instruments.
    D. handpieces.

99. The route of administration for drugs which enter directly into the lungs is known as (Ch. 10)
    A. intramuscular.
    B. inhalational.
    C. intravenous.
    D. intraosseous.

100. A written direction to a pharmacist to prepare a drug is called a (an) (Ch. 2)
    A. invoice.
    B. contract.
    C. prescription.
    D. order blank.

☑ answers to
practice exam

1.	A	26.	C	51.	B	76.	B
2.	D	27.	A	52.	D	77.	C
3.	A	28.	B	53.	A	78.	D
4.	B	29.	A	54.	D	79.	C
5.	B	30.	B	55.	C	80.	A
6.	C	31.	B	56.	C	81.	D
7.	B	32.	C	57.	B	82.	A
8.	B	33.	D	58.	E	83.	B
9.	D	34.	B	59.	B	84.	A
10.	B	35.	D	60.	B	85.	B
11.	C	36.	A	61.	C	86.	A
12.	A	37.	C	62.	D	87.	B
13.	D	38.	E	63.	E	88.	E
14.	D	39.	D	64.	B	89.	A
15.	B	40.	C	65.	A	90.	B
16.	B	41.	B	66.	C	91.	D
17.	B	42.	C	67.	D	92.	B
18.	A	43.	A	68.	B	93.	A
19.	A	44.	A	69.	A	94.	D
20.	C	45.	C	70.	B	95.	B
21.	C	46.	D	71.	D	96.	E
22.	D	47.	B	72.	C	97.	A
23.	C	48.	B	73.	A	98.	C
24.	D	49.	C	74.	B	99.	B
25.	B	50.	A	75.	C	100.	C

Glossary

Abrasion   the pathologic wearing away of tooth structure

Absorbent   capable of absorbing

Accessible   capable of being reached, used or seen

Acidic   of or pertaining to acid; acid-forming

Acute   a disorder or system that comes on suddenly, characterized by sharp or severe pain

ADA   American Dental Association

Adaptation   adjustment of an organism to a change in environment

Adhesion   the forces of attraction existing between two different objects or surfaces that hold them together

Adjacent   being close in proximity; meeting and touching at some point

Adversely   against or in contrary direction

Aerobe   microorganism that can live and grow only where free oxygen is present

Aerosol   particles of microscopic size dispensed in solution or suspended in air; dental aerosol is generated during use of dental armamentarium, for example, handpieces, sonics, air/water syringe

Agitate   shaking a container so that contents are mixed

AIDS   acquired immunodeficiency syndrome; the final stage of disease from the human immunodeficiency virus

Alkaline   of, relating to, containing, or having the properties of an alkali; especially a solution having a pH of more than 7

Allergy   hypersensitivity to a specific substance, for example, latex

Antibody   specialized protein produced in response to an antigen, creating an immunity

Antigen   substance that induces the formation of an immune response

Antimicrobial   capable of suppressing the growth of microorganisms

Antiseptic   compounds that inhibit the growth of bacteria

Apical   the apex or conical endings of the roots of the teeth

Armamentarium   the equipment and methods used especially in dentistry

Articulating   bones connected at joints

Asepsis   the absence of infection or pathogenic microorganisms

Aseptic   absence of pathogens

Asymptomatic   no symptoms of infection

Attrition   wearing or grinding down of the occlusal or incisal surfaces of teeth

Autoclave   an instrument for sterilization using moist heat under pressure

AZT   ZDV–Zibovudine-approved drug for initial therapy of primary HIV-1 infection

Bacteremia   presence of bacteria in the bloodstream

Bactericidal   a substance that destroys bacteria

Bacteriostatic   agent that stops the growth of bacteria

Barrier protection   protection against contamination provided by personal protective equipment

Beneficial   producing or promoting a favorable result; advantageous

Bioburden   microbial or organic material on an object prior to decontamination

Biohazard   contaminated substance that poses a biologic risk and potential for disease transmission

Biological indicator   monitoring device for heat and gas sterilizers, for example, vial containing endospores

Booster vaccination   vaccine injected at appropriate intervals after the primary immunization to sustain an immune response

Candidiasis   oral lesion associated with AIDS caused by the *Candida* species of yeastlike fungi

Caustic   any substance with a burning or corrosive action on body tissues

CDC   Centers for Disease Control and Prevention (CDCP)

Centric relation   a point determined when the mandible is in its most retruded position

Cephalometric   scientific measurement of the head

Chemical indicator   monitoring device for the process of checking temperature range during use of sterilizers, for example, autoclave striped tape, color change stripe on autoclave bags.

Chronic exposure   persisting over long period of time

Chronological age   arrangement in the order of occurence

Communicable   infectious; capable of being spread or transmitted

Condensation   the packing of filling materials into tooth cavities to eliminate voids within cavity or filling

Conscious sedation   a state of sedation in which the conscious patient is rendered free of fear, apprehension, and anxiety, through drugs

Contamination   introduction of blood or infectious agent on an item or surface

Contouring   to shape or form a surface as in carving a dental restoration

Convulsions   involuntary muscle contractions

Cross contamination   spread of disease through contact with contaminated items or surfaces

Cumulative effects   increasing by successive additions

Cyanoacrylate   toxic glue that is used as a tissue adhesive

Deactivate   the removal or loss of radioactivity from a previously radioactive material

Debridement   the removal of foreign material or tissue

Debris   soft foreign matter loosely attached to the surface of the tooth

Decontamination   use of physical or chemical means to destroy pathogens; removal of bioburden from surfaces

Deteriorate   impairment of mental or physical function; rot away

Developmental age   growth to full size or maturity as in tooth development

DHCW   dental health care worker

Diagnostic   distinctive of or serving as a criterion of a disease

Diastema   a space between two adjacent teeth in the same dental arch

Direct supervision   under the statutes of the state dental board defines performance of specific functions as being performed in the presence of the dentist

Discard   throw away; reject

Disengage   to sever or interrupt the connection of or between

Disinfectant   chemical agent applied to inanimate objects for the destruction of microorganisms; disinfectants do not destroy bacterial spores

Disinfection   the destruction or removal of pathogenic organisms by a chemical substance

Dislodge   to displace or force from a position

Dissipate   to vanish by dispersion

Distorted   twist out of a proper or natural relation of parts; misshape

Distract   to draw apart or divert

Droplet infection   disease transmission through small liquid droplets, as from sneezing and coughing

Edentulous   without teeth

Effective   a specific result measurable influence

Elective   a treatment or surgical procedure not requiring immediate attention, planned at patient's convenience

Elimination   excretion of waste products by the skin, kidneys, and intestines

ELISA   enzyme-linked immunosorbent assay; detection test for the presence of HIV antibody

Embedded   teeth that remain under the gums because there is not sufficient force to cause them to erupt

Embrasure   space formed by the contour and position of adjacent teeth

Endodontic   a branch of dentistry concerned with diagnosis, treatment, and prevention of diseases of the dental pulp and its surrounding tissues

Engineering controls   controls that isolate or remove the hazard from the workplace, for example, sharps disposal container

EPA   Environmental Protection Agency

Epidemic   rapid spreading of a disease among a population

Esthetic   of or concerning the appreciation of beauty or good taste

Evaporates   loss in volume due to conversion of a liquid into a vapor

Excessive   a quantity, an amount, or a degree that is more than what is justifiable

Exfoliate   the shedding of the primary set of teeth in man

Exposure control plan   a written plan required by OSHA that describes how exposure to bloodborne disease agents will be controlled at the workplace

Exposure incident   contact with infectious agent or blood during the performance of duties

External oblique   extending from the mental foramen, follows the length of the body of the mandible past the last tooth and up the ramus

External ventilation   outside circulation of fresh air into a room

Extracting   pulling out or removing teeth

Exudate   accumulation of a puslike fluid

Eye of needle   pointed instrument for suturing, eye is at tip

Facilitate   to make less difficult

FDA   Food and Drug Administration

Flush   irrigating of a cavity with water

Fungicidal   capable of killing fungi

Gingival related to the gums

Glove integrity strength and durability to resist tears and punctures, impervious to materials that will compromise use of gloves

Grating to grind the teeth together with a rasping sound.

Hairy leukoplakia oral lesion associated with HIV-positive infection; white in color, commonly found on lateral borders of tongue

Hazard communication standard OSHA law directing employers to provide employees with information on chemical hazards in the workplace

Hazardous waste contaminated waste which poses a biologic risk to the environment

HBIG hepatitis B immune globulin, prepared from plasma known to contain a high titer of antibody against HBsAg

HBV hepatitis B virus

HCW health care worker

Hematoma a swelling or mass of blood confined to an organ, tissue, or space and caused by a break in a blood vessel

Herringbone pattern pattern consisting of rows of short, slanted parallel lines with the direction of the slant alternating row by row

HIV human immunodeficiency virus

HIV+ seropositive indicates a positive test for the HIV antibody

Horizontal of or along the direction of the width

Host the organic body upon which or in which parasites live

Hyperventilation hyperpnea as occurs in forced respiration; increased inspiration and expiration of air as a result of increase in rate or depth of respiration

Immersion place under water or other solution

Immunity having antibodies to protect against a disease

Immunodeficiency inability of immune system to respond to an antigen

Impacted a tooth so placed in the jaw bone that eruption is impossible

Inadvertently unintentional due to oversight

Incipient beginning tooth decay

Incise to cut as with a sharp instrument

Incubation stage time between an infectious exposure and the appearance of signs and symptoms of disease

Infection condition in which the body is invaded by a pathogen

Infection control to control disease by performing specific procedures and eliminating the spread of contaminated agents

Infectious waste regulated waste contaminated with blood, saliva, or other infectious agents

Inhalation drawing in breath, gas or vapor into the lungs

Inhibit to hold back or keep from some action

Insoluble incapable of being dissolved, not soluble

Intact entire, unimpaired left whole

Interface to interact with another system, group, or discipline

Inter-maxillary between the maxillary structures

Intra-maxillary within the maxillary structures

Intrinsic due to causes from within the body

Invert to change to the direct opposite, reverse material

Kaposi's sarcoma oral lesion associated with HIV infection, malignant and of blood vessel origin

Latent to be hidden, undeveloped, unactive

Lateral toward the side, to position on the side

Leak to let a fluid substance out

Lethargy lack of energy, drowsiness

Luting to bind or hold together

Mastication chewing, grinding of food in the mouth

Medicament a medicine or remedy

Meticulous careful about details

Microbial growth cell division resulting in an increase in the number of cells

MMWR *Morbidity and Mortality Weekly Report* published by CDC

Mortician undertaker

Mottled condition in which the enamel of the teeth become discolored

MSDS material safety data sheet, which indicates chemical properties and hazards

Mulling to grind or pulverize

NIOSH National Institute for Occupational Safety and Health

Noncorrosive that which does not corrode, will not rust

Nullify to void or cancel out

Occlusal the chewing surface of posterior teeth premolars and molars

Occupational exposure reasonably anticipated skin, eye, mucous membrane, or parenteral contact with blood or other infectious materials that may result from the performance of an employee's duties

Opaque not transparent; impenetrable by visible light rays or x-ray

OPIM other potentially infectious materials

Opposing dentition the opposite dentition from the working arch, upper or lower arch

Oral cavity concerning the mouth

OSHA Occupational Safety and Health Administration

Parallel side by side; extending in the same direction and at the same point

Parenteral exposure as the result of breaking or piercing the skin barrier through events such as needlesticks, human bites, cuts, and abrasions

Particulate a very minute particle

Pathogen microorganism that is capable of causing a disease

Pathologic waste includes extracted teeth, biopsy specimens

Penetrates passes into, to enter or force into the interior

Percutaneous effected through the skin

Perpendicular at right angles to a given plane or line

Porosity the state of being porous; pores through which air, light, fluids may pass

Post-exposure evaluation follow-up report after an exposure incident given to the employee by the employer

Potentiates synergistic action of two substances which increases the potency or action

PPE personal protective equipment; specialized clothing or equipment worn by an employee for protection against a hazard, for example, gloves, mask, eyewear, uniforms, gowns, resuscitation bags, ventilation devices, face shields

Precise strictly defined, accurately stated

Promiscuous indiscriminate sexual behavior/activity

Prone opposite of supine, facing downward

Proximal nearest the point of attachment, side by side

psi pounds per square inch

Puncture wound wound made by piercing with sharp instrument

Radiolucent allowing x-rays to pass through

Radiopaque impenetrable to the x-ray or other forms of radiation

Recurrent returning at intervals

Regulated waste contaminated hazardous waste which requires OSHA disposal methods; includes liquid or semi-liquid blood or other potentially infectious materials

Replenish to make full or complete again, as by furnishing a new supply

Reposition to put into a new or different position

Reservoir bag holding device

Resorption degeneration of the root

Respiration inhaling, taking in oxygen and exhaling carbon dioxide

Restriction kept within certain limits

Rigid not bending or flexible

Secondary container a container which is not considered primary, often used for transfer

Sepsis presence of infectious disease-producing microorganisms

Sharps objects capable of penetrating the skin, for example, needles, broken glass

Sharps container puncture-resistant container for the disposal of needles, scalpel blades, ortho wires, or other sharp items

Shelf life storage time period of a product before activation or use which denotes that it will still retain effectiveness

Simultaneously existing together or at the same time

Slurry thin, watery mixture such as plaster slurry

Solvent a substance that dissolves another substance

Source individual any individual, living or dead, whose blood or other potentially infectious materials may be a source of occupational exposure to the employee

Spatulation spreading or blending substances with a spatula

Sporicide agent capable of killing spores

Stablize to make steady or firm, to secure

Sterilant an agent capable of killing all microorganisms

Sterilization the removal or destruction of all microorganisms

Stippling pitted appearance seen on attached gingiva

Subsequent to follow close after

Supine reclining position of patient

Surface asepsis procedures that prevent the spread of infectious agents on environmental surfaces

Syncope fainting

Synergistic phenolics harmonious action of two chemical disinfectants

Tease to separate into minute parts

Tensible materials capability of being stretched

Thermal sensitivity capacity for the recognition of heat

Toxic pertaining to a poison or toxin

Toxic waste waste which is poisonous or toxic

Translucent not transparent but permitting the passage of light

Transmission a transfer from one individual to another

Trismus tonic contraction of the muscles of mastication

Trituration homogenous mixture of metal alloy particles and mercury to form dental amalgam

Tuberculocide agent that can kill *Mycobacterium tuberculosis*

Unit dosing units used to define measurement or radiation relative to dose, dose equivalent and exposure

Universal precautions considering all patients as being infected with pathogens; therefore applying infection control procedures to all patients

Use life time period a solution is effective after activation or preparation

User a person or thing that uses

Vaccination the production of immunity to a specific disease by placing a vaccine into the body

Vaccine substance that contains an antigen to which the immune system can respond

Verification confirmation of the truth

Versus in contrast with

Vertical upright; straight up or down

Virucidal agent that kills viruses

Virus submicroscopic organism which causes infectious diseases

Zibovudine AZT/ZDV approved drug for initial therapy of primary HIV-1 infection

Bibliography

American Dental Assistants Association Department of Continuing Education. *ICE PACK.* 1998.

American Heart Association. *BLS for Healthcare Providers,* American Heart Association National Center. Dallas, Texas: 2001.

American Red Cross. *American Red Cross Standard First Aid Workbook.* 1991.

American Red Cross. *Advanced First Aid and Emergency Care,* 2nd ed. New York: Doubleday and Co., Inc., 1980.

Anthony CP, Thibodeau GA. *Structure and Function of the Body,* 8th ed. St. Louis: CV Mosby Co., 1988.

Atchison KA. *Radiographic Safety.* Western Dental Education Center Correspondence Course. Los Angeles: Department of Veterans Affairs, West Los Angeles VA Medical Center, 1987.

Boucher CO. *Boucher's Clinical Dental Terminology: Glossary of Accepted Terms in All Disciplines of Dentistry,* 4th ed. St. Louis: CV Mosby Co., 1993.

Brand R. Isselhard, D. *Anatomy of Oral Facial Structures,* 6th ed. St. Louis: Mosby, Inc., 1998.

Brown SK. *Infection Control in Dental Practices.* Miami, FL: Health Studies Institute, Inc., 1993.

Butsumyo D, Deboom G, Lynne S, Parrot K. *Principles and Practice of Dental Radiography.* Los Angeles: Western Dental Education Center Correspondence Course. Department of Veterans Affairs, West Los Angeles VA Medical Center, 1988.

Caplan CM. *Dental Practice Management Encyclopedia.* Penn Well, 1985.

Carter C, Bishop J, Kravits SL. *Keys To Effective Learning,* 2nd ed. Upper Saddle River NJ: Prentice Hall Inc., 2000.

Carter LM, Yaman P, Ladley BA, Eds. *Dental Instruments.* St. Louis: CV Mosby Co., 1981.

Chasteen JE, Cara Miyasaki Ching, *Essentials of Clinical Dental Assisting,* 5th ed. St. Louis: CV Mosby Co., 1997.

Chen PS. *Chemistry: Inorganic, Organic and Biological,* 2nd ed. New York: Harper & Row Publishers Inc., 1980.

Chernega JB, *Emergency Guide for Dental Auxiliaries,* 3rd ed. Albany, New York: Delmar, 2002.

Christensen GJ. Glass Ionomer as a Luting Material. *J Am Dent Assoc.* 1990; 120: 55–57.

Ciancio SG, Bourgault PC. *Clinical Pharmacology for Dental Professionals,* 3rd ed. Chicago: Year Book Medical Publishers, Inc., 1989.

Cochran DL, Klakwarf K, Brunsvold M. *Plaque and Calculus Removal Considerations for the Professional.* Chicago: Quintessence Publishing Co., Inc., 1994.

Cottone JA, Molinari JA, Terezhalmy G. *Practical Infection Control in Dentistry,* 2nd ed. Mavern, PA: Lea & Febiger, 1996.

Craig RG. *Restorative Dental Materials,* 9th ed. St Louis: CV Mosby Co., 1993.

Craig RG, Hon, Powers JM, Wataha JC. *Dental Materials Properties and Manipulation,* 7th ed., Harcourt Health Sciences W.B. Saunders, Mosby, Churchill Livingstone. 2000.

Cuny E. Fredekind R. (2002) *OSHA Bloodborne Pathogens Rule,* Compendium of Continuing Education in Dentistry, Vol. 23, No. 3.

Davis K. *Training Manual for Oral and Maxillofacial Surgery Assistants,* 3rd ed. Lomita, CA: King Printing, 1996.

deLyre WR, Johnson N. *Essentials of Dental Radiology for Dental Assistants and Hygienists,* 5th ed. Stamford, CT: Appleton & Lange, 1995.

DePaola LG, Carpenter WM. (2002) *Bloodborne Pathogens: Current Concepts,* Compendium of Continuing Education in Dentistry, Vol. 23, No.3.

Dietz E, Badavinac R. *Safety Standards and Infection Control for Dental Hygienists,* Albany, New York: Delmar, 2002.

Domer LR, Snyder TL, Heid DW, Eds. *Dental Practice Management.* St. Louis: CV Mosby Co., 1980.

Eastman Kodak Company. *Successful Panoramic Radiography.* Rochester, NY, 1998.

Eastman Kodak Company. *Quality Assurance in Dental Radiography.* Rochester, NY, 1996.

Eastman Kodak Company. *Radiation Safety in Dental Radiography.* Rochester, NY, 1998.

Eastman Kodak Company. *X-rays in Dentistry.* Rochester, NY, 1985.

Ehrlich A. *Business Administration for the Dental Assistant,* 4th ed. Champaign, IL: Colwell Systems, 1991.

Ehrlich A. *Nutrition and Dental Health, 2nd ed.* Albany, NY: Delmar Publications, 1994.

Facts About AIDS for the Dental Team, 3rd ed. American Dental Association Council on Dental Therapeutics, Chicago: American Dental Association, October 1991.

Ferracane JL. *Materials in Dentistry Principles and Applications,* 2nd ed. Baltimore, MD: Lippincott Williams & Wilkins, 2001.

Finkbeiner BL, Johnson CS. *Comprehensive Dental Assisting.* St. Louis: CV Mosby Co., 1998.

Finkbeiner BL, Finkbeiner CA. *Practice Management for the Dental Team,* 5th ed. St. Louis: CV Mosby Co., 2001.

Frommer HH. *Radiology for Dental Auxiliaries,* 7th ed. St. Louis: CV Mosby Co., 2000.

Fuller JL, Denehy GE. *Concise Dental Anatomy and Morphology,* 4th ed. Chicago: Year Book Medical Publishers, Inc., 2001.

Gilmore, HW, et al. *Operative Dentistry,* 4th ed. St. Louis: CV Mosby Co., 1982.

Giunta JL. *Oral Pathology,* 3rd ed. Philadelphia: BC Decker, Inc., 1989.

Gladwin M. Bagby M. *Clinical Aspects of Dental Materials,* Baltimore, MD: Lippincott Williams & Wilkins, 2000.

Goss CM. *Gray's Anatomy,* 37th ed. Philadelphia: Lea & Febiger Publishers, 1989.

Goth A. *Medical Pharmacology,* 13th ed. St. Louis: CV Mosby Co., 1992.

Guthrie HA. *Human Nutrition.* St. Louis: CV Mosby Co., 1995.

Haring JI, Jansen L. *Dental Radiograhy Principles and Techniques,* 2nd ed. Philadelphia, W.B.Saunders Co., 2000.

Harris NO, Garcia-Godoy F. *Primary Preventive Dentistry,* 5th ed. Upper Saddle River, NJ: Prentice Hall Health, 1999.

Hefferson JJ, Ayer WA, Koehler HM, Eds. *Foods, Nutrition and Dental Health,* Vol. I. South, IL: Pathodox Publishers, 1980.

Hiatt JL, Gartner LP, *Textbook of Head and Neck Anatomy,* 3rd ed. Baltimore, MD: Lippincott Williams & Wilkins 2001.

Hooley J, Whitacre R. *Medications Used in Oral Surgery,* 3rd ed. Seattle: Stoma Press, Inc, 1984.

Infection Control in the Dental Environment. Department of Veterans Affairs, American Dental Association, Department of Health and Human Services and Centers for Disease Control. Washington, DC: Eastern Dental Education Center Learning Resources Center, Veterans Administration, 1989.

Jawetz E, et al. *Review of Medical Microbiology,* 20th ed. Stamford, CT: Appleton & Lange, 1995.

Keeton WT. *Biological Science,* 6th ed. New York: WW Norton and Co., 1996.

Kumar, Angell M. Robbins. *Basic Pathology,* 7th ed. Philadelphia: WB Saunders Co., 2002.

Ladley BA, Wilson SA. *Review of Dental Assisting.* St. Louis: CV Mosby Co., 1980.

Langland OE. *Radiography for Dental Hygienists & Dental Assistants,* 3rd ed. Springfield, IL: Charles C Thomas Publishers, 1988.

Langland OE, Langlais RP, Preece JW. *Principles of Dental Imaging* 2nd ed. Baltimore, MD: Lippincott Williams & Wilkins 2002.

Little JW, Falace DA. *Dental Management of the Medically Compromised Patient,* 5th ed. St. Louis: CV Mosby Co., 1997.

Malamed SF. *Medical Emergencies in the Dental Office,* 5th ed. St. Louis: CV Mosby Co., 2000.

Manson-Hing LR. *Fundamentals of Dental Radiography,* 3rd ed. Philadelphia: Lea & Febiger Publishers, 1990.

Miles D, Van Dis M, Jensen C, Ferretti A. *Radiographic Imaging for Dental Auxiliaries,* 3rd ed. Philadelphia: WB Saunders Co., 1999.

Miller BF, Keane CB. *Encyclopedia and Dictionary of Medicine, Nursing, and Allied Health,* 6th ed. Philadelphia: WB Saunders Co., 1997.

Miller CH, Palenik CJ. *Infection Control and Management of Hazardous Materials for the Dental Team.* 2nd ed. St. Louis: CV Mosby Co., 1998.

Miller F. *College Physics,* 6th ed. New York: Harcourt Brace Jovanovich, Inc, 1987.

Muma RD, Lyons B, Borucki MJ, Pollard RB. *HIV Manual for Health Care Professionals.* Stamford, 2nd ed. CT: Appleton & Lange, 1997.

Newman HN. *Dental Plaque.* Springfield, IL: Charles C Thomas Publishers, 1980.

Olson S. *Dental Radiography Laboratory Manual.* Philadelphia: WB Saunders Co., 1995.

Orban B. *Oral History and Embryology,* 11th ed. St. Louis: CV Mosby Co., 1991.

Organization for Safety and Asepsis Procedures (02/2002) *Postexposure Management,* Monthly Focus, Annapolis, MD.

Organization for Safety and Asepsis Procedures (Pub. No. 4-2001) *Sharps Safety & OSHA Compliance,* Monthly Focus, Annapolis, MD.

Organization for Safety and Asepsis Procedures (Pub. No. 5-2001) *Handpiece Sterilization & Maintenance,* Monthly Focus, Annapolis, MD.

Organization for Safety and Asepsis Procedures (Pub. No. 8-2001) *Environmental Surface Asepsis,* Monthly Focus, Annapolis, MD.

Organization for Safety and Asepsis Procedures (Focus #2-2000) *MSDSs, Chemical Lists & Other HazCom Musts,* Monthly Focus, Annapolis, MD.

Organization for Safety and Asepsis Procedures (Focus #3-2000) *Selecting & Evaluating a Sterilization Monitoring Service,* Monthly Focus, Annapolis, MD.

Peterson LJ. *Contemporary Oral and Maxillofacial Surgery,* 3rd ed. St. Louis: CV Mosby Co., 1998.

Philips RW. Moore B.K. *Elements of Dental Materials for Dental Hygienists and Assistants,* 6th ed. Philadelphia: WB Saunders Co., 1998.

Phinney DJ, Halstead JH. *Dental Assisting A Comprehensive Approach,* 1st ed. Albany, New York: Delmar, 2000.

Randolph PM, Dennison CI. *Diet, Nutrition, and Dentistry.* St. Louis: CV Mosby Co., 1981.

Richardson RE, Barton RE. *The Dental Assistant,* 6th ed. New York: McGraw-Hill Inc, 1988.

Rose LF, Kaye D. *Internal Medicine for Dentistry,* 2nd ed. St. Louis: CV Mosby Co., 1990.

Rowe AHR, Alexander AG. *Clinical Methods, Medicine, Pathology and Pharmacology—A Companion to Dental Studies,* Vol 2. Boston: Blackwell Scientific Publications, 1988.

Sande MA, Volberding PA. *The Medical Management of AIDS,* 6th ed. Philadelphia: WB Saunders Co., 1999.

Schwarzrock SP, Jensen JR. *Effective Dental Assisting,* 7th ed. Dubuque, IA: William C Brown Co., 1991.

Section on Instructional System Design, Department of Periodontology, School of Dentistry, University of California, San Francisco. Plaque Control Instruction. Berkeley, CA: Praxis Publishing Co., 1978.

Seymour RA, Walton JG. *Adverse Drug Reactions in Dentistry.* 2nd ed. New York: Oxford University Press, 1996.

Shafer WG, Hine MK, Levy BM. *Textbook of Oral Pathology,* 4th ed. Philadelphia: WB Saunders Co., 1983.

Shannon Mills CE. Karpay RI. (2002) *Dental Waterlines and Biofilm,* Compendium of Continuing Education in Dentistry, Vol. 23, No. 3.

Shin D, Avers J. *AIDS/HIV Reference Guide for Medical Professionals.* West Los Angeles, CA: CIRID/UCLA School of Medicine Publishers, 1988.

Sicher H. *Sicher's Oral Anatomy,* 8th ed. St. Louis: CV Mosby Co., 1988.

Skinner EW, Philips RW. *Skinner's Science of Dental Materials,* 9th ed. Philadelphia: WB Saunders Co., 1991.

Smith DC. Dental Cements. *Adv Dent Res.* 1988; 2:134–141.

Spohn EE, Halouski WA, Berry TC. *Operative Dentistry Procedures for Dental Auxiliaries.* St. Louis: CV Mosby Co., 1981.

Stedman's Concise Medical Dictionary for the Health Professions Illustrated, 4th ed. Hagerstown, MD: Lippincott Williams & Wilkins, 2001.

Supplement—Handling Hazardous Chemicals General Guidelines, American Dental Association, 1995.

Suzuki M, Jordan R. Glass Ionomer—Composite Sandwich Technique. *J Am Dent Assoc.* 1990; 120:55–57.

Taber's Cyclopedic Medical Dictionary. 17th ed. Philadelphia: F.A. Davis Company, 1993.

Thibodeau GA. *Anatomy and Physiology,* 4th ed. St. Louis: CV Mosby Co., 1999.

Torres H, Ehrlich A, Bird D, Dietz E. *Modern Dental Assisting,* 6th ed. Philadelphia: WB Saunders Co., 1999.

Tyldesley WR. *Oral Medicine,* 4th ed. New York: Oxford University Press, 1995.

U.S. Department of Labor, Office of Health Compliance Assistance. OSHA Hazard Communication Standard, *Code of Federal Regulations, #29,* Part 1910 et al., Feburary 9, 1994.

U.S. Department of Labor, Occupational Safety and Health Administration. *Controlling Occupational Exposure to Bloodborne Pathogens in Dentistry.* OSHA Publication 3129, 1996.

U.S. Department of Labor, Occupational Safety and Health Administration. *Chemical Hazard Communication.* OSHA Publication 3084 (Revised), 1994.

U.S. Department of Labor, Occupational Safety and Health Administration. *Hazard Communication Guidelines for Compliance.* OSHA Publication 3111, 2000.

U.S. Department of Labor, Occupational Safety and Health Administration. *All About OSHA,* OSHA 2056 (Revised 2000).

Veterans Administration Medical Center. *Periodontal Resident Manual.* West Los Angeles, CA: VA Medical Center, 1990.

Wheeler S. *Dental Anatomy, Physiology and Occlusion,* 7th ed. Philadelphia: WB Saunders Co., 1992.

Wheeler S. *An Atlas of Tooth Form,* 5th ed. Philadelphia: WB Saunders Co., 1984.

Wilkins EM. *Clinical Practice of the Dental Hygienist,* 8th ed. Philadelphia: Lea & Febiger, 1999.

Woodall IR. *Legal, Ethical, and Management Aspects of the Dental Care System,* 3rd ed. St. Louis: CV Mosby Co., 1987.

Woelfel, JB., Scheid RC. *Dental Anatomy It's Relevance to Dentistry,* 6th ed. Hagerstown, MD: Lippincott Williams & Wilkins, 2001.

Wuehrmann A, Manson-Hing LR. *Dental Radiology,* 5th ed. St. Louis: CV Mosby Co., 1981.

Zwemer TJ. *Boucher's Clinical Dental Terminology,* 4th ed. St. Louis: CV Mosby Co., 1993.

Resources for Further Information

American Academy of General Dentistry
211 East Chicago Avenue
Suite 1200
Chicago, Illinois 60611-2670
312-4404300
www.agd.org

American Academy of Periodontology
737 North Michigan Avenue
Suite 800
Chicago, Illinois 60611-2690
312-787-5518
www.perio.org

American Association of Orthodontists
401 N. Lindberg
St. Louis, Missouri 63141-7816
314-993-1700
www.aaortho.org

American Dental Assistants Association
203 North LaSalle Street
Chicago, Illinois 60601-1225
312-541-1550
www.adaa.org

American Dental Association (ADA)
211 E. Chicago Avenue
Chicago, Illinois 60611
312-440-2500
www.ada.org

American Heart Association
7320 Greenville Avenue
Dallas, Texas 75231
www.americanheart.org

Centers for Disease Control and Prevention (CDC)
National Center of Infectious Diseases
1600 Clifton Road, NE
Atlanta, Georgia 30333
404-639-3311
www.cdc.gov

Dental Assisting National Board, Inc.
676 North Saint Clair, Suite 1880
Chicago, Illinois 60611
1-800-367-3262
www.danb.org

Environmental Protection Agency (EPA)
National United States
www.epa.gov

Food and Drug Administration (FDA)
Office of Consumer Affairs
5600 Fisher's Lane
Rockville, Maryland 20857
301-827-4420
www.fda.gov

Office of Sterilization and Asepsis Procedures (OSAP)
Research Foundation
P.O. Box 6297
Annapolis, Maryland 21401
800-298-6727
www.osap@clark.net

National Institute of Dental and Craniofacial Research
Building 31 Room2C35
31 Center Drive MSC-2290
Bethesda, Maryland 20892-2290
301-496-4261
www.nidr.nih.gov/

National Institute for Occupational Safety and Health
(NIOSH)
4676 Columbus Parkway,
Cincinnati, Ohio 45226
1-800-356-4674
www.cdc.gov/niosh

Occupational Safety and Health Administration (OSHA)
Main Office
200 Constitution Avenue
NW, Washington DC 20210
202-219-7242
www.osha.gov

Index

A

Abrasive dental materials, 108
Accounts receivable/payable management, 168–170
Acid etchants, 139
Acquired immunodeficiency syndrome (AIDS), 22
Acrylic resins, dental materials, 103
   denture based, 107
Acute necrotizing ulcerative gingivitis (ANUG), 20
Aerosol, 114
ALARA, 74
Alginate, 106
Allergies, 148
Anatomic landmarks of the skull, 32
   cranium, 32
   mandible, 32
   maxilla, 32
Antibiotics, 23
Appointment book/day sheet, management of, 167–168
Arteries, 16
Articulations, 15
Artifical respiration, medical emergencies, 152–153
Asepsis, 116
Autoimmune disorders, 22
Axial skeleton, 14

B

Bacterial plaque, 48
Barrier techniques, infection control, 115
Bilogical monitoring, 118
Biohazard, 130
Biomedical sciences, 13–29
   autoimmune disorders, 22
   cytology and histology, 18
   dental caries, 20–21
   lesions associated with infectious diseases, 22–23
   microbiology, 18–19
   oral pathologic conditions, 21–22
   oral pathology, 19
   periodontium, diseases of, 20
   pharmacology, 23–25
   systems of the body, 14–15
      circulatory, 16
      digestive, 16
      endocrine, 17–18
      excretory, 17
      lymphatic, 16
      muscular, 15
      nervous, 15
      reproductive, 18
      respiratory, 16
      skeletal, 14–15
Bisecting, 84
Bitewing radiographs, 78
Bleaching agents, dental materials, 105
Bleeding disorders, medical emergencies, 157
Bloodborne pathogens exposure, controlling, 128–129
Bloodborne pathogen standard, 128
Bonding agents, 103
Bone marrow, 14
Brachial artery, 149

C

Calcification, 37
Calculus, 49

Canines, 37
Cardiopulmonary resuscitation (CPR), 150
Cardiovascular emergency, 153–154
Carotid artery, 149
Cast gold restorations, dental materials, 107
Cements in dentistry, 104–105
    glass ionomer, 104
    polycarboxylate, 104–105
    zinc-oxide eugenol (ZOE), 104
    zinc phosphate, 104
Cerebrovascular accident (CVA), 156
Certified Dental Assistant Candidate's Guide, 2
Certified Dental Assisting Examination, 1–11, 177–187
    administration of, 2
    distribution of items, 3–4
        chairside component, 4
        infection control component, 4
        radiation health and safety component, 4
    eligibility requirements, 2
    examination format, 3
    examination scoring, 10–11
    multiple choice test strategies, 8–9
    physical conditions during, 11
    simulated comprehensive exam, 177–187
    test anxiety, 9
    testing candidates with disabilities, 3
    testing schedule, 3
    types of questions, 4–8
        complex multiple choice, 7–8
        matching, 6–7
        negative format, 6
        single-item, 4–6
Certified Dental Practice Management Administrator
    (CDPMA) examination, 3
Certified Orthodontic Assistant (COA) examination, 3
Chairside assisting, 59–69
    charting, 62–63
    dental specialties, 63–65
    seating the patient, 60
    transfering instruments, 60–61
    zones of operating activity, 60
Charting, chairside assisting, 62–63
Choking, medical emergencies, 156
Circulatory system, 16
Collimation, 73
Complex multiple-choice questions, 7–8
Composite resins, 103
Confidentiality, 167
Consultation, 167
Contrast, 76
Convulsive disorders, medical emergencies, 156
Coronary heart disease (CHD), 153
Cranial nerves, 15
Cranium, 32
    bones of, table, 34
Credit charge, 168

Credits, 170
Custom trays, dental materials, 107
Cyanosis, 154
Cytology, 18

D
Debit charge, 168
Debits, 170
Decontamination, 119
Density, 76
Dental anatomy, 31–46
    anatomic landmarks of the skull, 32
    major muscles, 35–37
    occlusion, 39–41
    oral embryology, 37
    periodontium, 41–42
    salivary glands, 32–35
    soft tissue landmarks of the oral cavity, 32
    tongue, 35
    tooth morphology, 37–39
Dental Assisting National Board, Inc. (DANB), 2
Dental caries, 20–21
Dental floss/flossing technique, 50
Dental implants, 65
Dental laboratory disinfection, 119
Dental materials, 99–112
    abrasive, 108
    acrylic denture base resins, 107
    acrylic resins, 103
    bleaching agents, 105
    bonding agents, 103
    cast gold restorations, 107
    cements in dentistry, 104–105
    composite resin materials, 103
    custom trays, 107
    elastic impression materials, 106–107
    elastomeric impression materials, 105–106
    endodontic sedative/palliative, 108
    gypsum products: plaster and stone, 100–101
    pit-and-fissure sealants, 103
    plastic impression materials, 107
    porcelain, 105
    properties of matter, 100
    restorative materials used for permanent restorations,
        101–103
    varnishes/liners, 105
Dental office general/product safety guidelines, 139–141
Dental practice management, 163–176
    accounts receivable/payable, 168–170
    appointment book/day sheet, 167–168
    inventory systems, 171
    office manual, 164–165
    patient reception, 167
    patient records, 167
    personnel management, 165
    recall (recare) system, 168

record/bookeeping systems, 167
telephone communication, 165–166
third-party carriers, 170–171
Dental sealants, 51
Dental specialties, 63–65
endodontics, 64
oral/maxillofacial surgery, 64
oral pathology, 64
orthodontics, 64–65
pedodontics, 65
periodontics, 65
prosthodontics, 65
public health, 64
Dental stains, 48
Detoxifies, 17
Development process, 89–91
Diastolic, 149
Digestive system, 16
Disability conditions, testing candidates with, 3
Disclosing agent, 50
Disease transmission, modes of, 114
Disinfection, infection control, 118–119
Drug-induced medical emergency, 157

E
Elastic impression materials, dental materials, 106–107
Elastomeric, 105–106
impression materials, dental materials, 105–106
Employee communication program, 132–134
Endocrine system, 17–18
Endodontics, 64
Endodontic sedative/palliative dental materials, 108
Endothermic, 100
Engineering controls, occupational safety, 129
Examination format, Dental Assisting Certification exam, 3
Examination items, distribution of, 3–4
chairside component, 4
infection control component, 4
radiation health and safety component, 4
specialty examinations, 4
Examination scoring, 10–11
Excretory system, 17
Exfoliate, 37
Exothermic, 100
Exposing radiographs, rules for, 86–89
Exposure control plan, occupational safety, 131
Exposures, radiograph, 75–76
Exposure time, 73
Extraoral films, 78–80
Extrinsic stains, 48
Eyewash station, 132

F
Face, bones of, table, 34
Facsimile (fax), 166

Film badges, 75
Fixer, 90
Fluoride, 50–51
topical fluoride characteristics, table, 51
Focal-film distances (FFDs), 76

G
Gypsum, 100
products: plaster and stone, 100–101

H
Handwashing, infection control, 116
Hard deposits, 49
calculus, 49
formation of calculus, 49
Hazard communication standard, occupational safety, 135
Hepatitis B vaccination, 114, 131
Histology, 18
Homeostasis, 15
Hormones, 17
Housekeeping, occupational safety, 130
Human immunodeficiency virus (HIV), 128
Hyperventilation, 151
Hypnotics, 23
Hypotension, 149

I
Imbibition, 106
Immunization, 114
Incisors, 37
Infection control, 113–125
barrier techniques, 115
dental laboratory disinfection, 119
disease transmission, modes of, 114
disinfection, 118–119
handwashing, 116
hepatitis B vaccination, 114
management of office waste, 121
medical history data, 114
personal protective equipment (PPE), 115
post-treatment, 119–120
pre-treatment, 119
radiation asepsis, 121
sterilization, 116–118
monitoring, 118
preparing dental instruments for, 120–121
universal (standard) precautions, 114
Infection control and radiographs, 92–93
Informed consent, 167
Intermediate-level disinfection, 118
Interproximal brush, 50
Intraoral radiographs, 78
Intraoral radiography, techniques of, 84–86
Intrinsic stains, 49
Inventory systems, 171
Inverse square law, 74

K

Key nutrients, table, 52
Kilovolt peak (kvp), 73

L

Labeling, occupational safety, 135
Laundry, occupational safety, 131
Lesions associated with infectious diseases, 22–23
Light cure, 104
Lymphadenopathy, 16
Lymphatic system, 16
Lymphocytes, 16

M

Malocclusion, 64
Mandible, 32
Matching questions, 6–7
Materia alba, 48
Material safety data sheet (MSDS), 135–137
Matter, properties of, 100
Maxilla, 32
Maxillofacial surgery, 64
Medical emergencies, 147–161
    artifical respiration, 152–153
    bleeding disorders, 157
    cardiovascular emergency, 153–154
    cerebrovascular accident (CVA), 156
    choking, 156
    convulsive disorders, 156
    drug-induced emergencies, 157
    medical history, 148
    metabolic disorders, 156
    office preparation, 150–151
    postural hypotension (orthostatic hypotension), 155–156
    respiratory emergencies, 151–152
    shock, 154
    syncope, 155
    vital signs, 148–150
Medical history data, infection control, 114
Mercury toxicity, 103
Metabolic disorders, medical emergency, 156
Microbiology, 18–19
Millamperage (ma), 73
Molars, 37
Monomer, 103
Mottled enamel, 49
Mounting radiographs, 91–92
Multiple-choice test strategies, 8–9
Muscular system, 15

N

National Organization for Competency Assurance
        (NOCA), 2
Negative format questions, 6
Nervous system, 15
Non-narcotic analgesics, 23
Nutrients, 51

Nutrition/diet analysis, 51–53
    six key nutrient groups, 51

O

Obturation, 64
Occlusion, 39–41
Occupational safety, 127–146
    bloodborne pathogen exposure, controlling, 128–129
    bloodborne pathogen standard, 128
    dental office general/product safety guidelines, 139–141
    employee communication program, 132–134
    engineering controls, 129
    exposure control plan, 131
    exposure incident follow-up, 132
    hazard communication standard, 135
    hepatitis b vaccination, 131
    housekeeping, 130
    labeling, 135
    laundry, 131
    material safety data sheets, 135
    record keeping, 131
    training/employee information, 138
    waste handling, 130–131
    work practice controls, 129–130
    written hazard communication program, 138
Office manual, 164–165
Office preparation, medical emergencies, 150–151
Office waste, management of, infection control, 121
Oral cavity
    muscles in, 35–37
    soft tissue landmarks, 32
Oral embryology, 37
Oral pathologic conditions, 21–22
Oral pathology, 19, 64
Oral physiotherapy devices, 50
Oral surgery, 64
Orthodontics, 64–65
OSHA, 128

P

Panoramic radiography, 81–84
    advantages of, 81–82
    common errors in, 83–84
    disadvantages of, 82–83
Parasympathetic, 15
Pathogens, 116
Patient reception, 167
Patient records, 167
Pedodontics, 65
Periapical radiographs, 78
Periodontics, 65
Periodontium, 41–42
    diseases of, 20
Personal protective equipment (PPE), 115
Personnel management, 165
Pharmacology, 23–25
Pit-and-fissure sealants, 103

Plaque control programs, 54
Plaque formation, 48
Plastic impression, dental materials, 107
Platelets, 16
Polymer, 103
Polymerization, 103
Porcelain, dental, 105
Post treatment infection control, 119–120
Postural hypotension (orthostatic hypotension), 155–156
Premolars, 37
Pre-treatment infection control, 119
Preventive dentistry, 47–58
    dental floss/flossing technique, 50
    dental sealants, 51
    fluorides, 50–51
    hard deposits, 49
    nutrition/diet analysis, 51–53
    oral physiotherapy devices, 50
    plaque control programs, 54
    toothbrushes and brushing techniques, 49
Primary radiation, 72
Prosthodontics, 65
Ptyalin, 17
Public health, dental specialties, 64

Q
Quadrants, 63

R
Radiation, 72–75, 121
    asepsis, infection control, 121
    effects and safety, 74
    limits for operators, 74
    primary, 72
    protection guidelines, 74
    protective measures for, 74
    secondary, 73
    short- and long-term effects of, 74
Radiographs, 75–76, 78, 86, 89–93
    development process of, 89–91
    exposures, 75–76
    extraoral films, 78–80
    full-series surveys of, 86
    infection control and, 92–93
    intraoral, 78
        techniques of, 84–86
    rules for exposing, 86–89
    steps for mounting, 91–92
Radiology, 71–97
    basic principles of, 72–73
    extraoral films, 78–80
    film packet, 76–77
    panoramic radiography, 81–84
    radiation effects and safety, 74–75
    radiographic exposures, 75–76
Radiolucent, 75
Radiopaque, 75

Recall (recare)
    appointment, 54
    system, 168
Receipt, 170
Reconcile, 170
Recordkeeping, occupational safety, 131
Red blood cells, 16
Reimburse, 170
Reproductive system, 18
Respiration, 16
Respiratory, medical emergencies, 151–152
Respiratory system, 16
Restorative materials used for permanent restorations, 101–103

S
Saliva, 17
Salivary glands, 32–35
Sealants, 51
Seating the patient, chairside assisting, 60
Secondary radiation, 73
Sedation, 64
Sedatives, 23
Sepsis, 116
Shock, medical emergencies, 154
Simulated comprehensive exam, 177–187
Single-item questions, 4–6
Skeletal system, 14–15
Soft deposits, 48–49
    bacterial plaque, 48
    dental stains, 48
    materia alba, 48
    stages of plaque formation, 48
Source individual, 132
Sphygmomanometer, 149
Sporicidal, 118
Standard full series radiograph surveys, 86
Sterilization, infection control, 116–118, 120–121
    monitoring, 118
    preparing dental instruments for, 120–121
Succedaneous teeth, 37
Sulcus, 49
Sympathetic, 15
Syncope, medical emergencies, 155
Syneresis, 106
Systems of the body, 14–15
    circulatory, 16
    digestive, 16
    endocrine, 17–18
    excretory, 17
    lymphatic, 16
    muscular, 15
    nervous, 15
    reproductive, 18
    respiratory, 16
    skeletal, 14–15
Systolic, 148

T
Telephone communication, 165–166
Temporomandibular joint, 32
Test anxiety, 9–10
Testing schedule, 3
Third-party carriers, 170–171
Tongue, 35
Toothbrush/brushing techniques, 49
Tooth morphology, 37–39
Training/employee information, occupational safety, 138
Transferring instruments, chairside assisting, 60–61
Trendelenburg position, 155
Trigeminal nerve, 37
Trituration, 101
Tuberculocidal, 118

U
Universal precautions, 114

V
Varnishes/liners, dental materials, 105
Vasodilators, 151

Veins, 16
Vital signs, medical emergencies, 148–150

W
Waste handling, occupational safety, 130–131
White blood cells, 16
Work practice controls, occupational safety, 129–130
Written exposure control plan, 131
Written hazard communication program, occupational safety, 138

X
X-rays, 72
    characteristics of, 72
    film packets, 76–77
    production of, necessary components, 72
    unit parameters controlled by operator, 73